PRESCRIPTION AND NONPRESCRIPTION MEDICATIONS FOR Children

PRESCRIPTION AND NONPRESCRIPTION MEDICATIONS FOR Children

WHAT PARENTS NEED TO KNOW

MAX VAN GILDER, M.D. AND
SHELAGH RYAN MASLINE

A LYNN SONBERG BOOK

POCKET BOOKS
New York London Toronto Sydney Tokyo Singapore

An *Original* Publication of POCKET BOOKS

POCKET BOOKS, a division of Simon & Schuster Inc.
1230 Avenue of the Americas, New York, NY 10020

Published by arrangement with:

Lynn Sonberg Book Associates
10 West 86th Street
New York, NY 10024

ISBN: 0-671-51069-X

First Pocket Books printing July 1997

10 9 8 7 6 5 4 3 2 1

Text design by Stanley S. Drate/Folio Graphics Co. Inc.

Printed in the U.S.A.

IMPORTANT NOTE: This book was written to provide selected information to the public concerning prescription and over-the-counter medications for children. Research about these drugs is an ongoing process; side effects and adverse reactions to particular drugs sometimes continue to be reported to the FDA after a drug has been approved for use in the general market. While every effort has been made to include the most up-to-date information in this book, there can be no guarantee that what we know about these medications won't change with time and further research. Readers should bear in mind that this book is not intended to be used to help parents diagnose or treat their children. Parents should consult a pediatrician or other appropriate health professional regarding all medical problems. Readers should never stop giving their children a prescription drug or alter the dosage or dosing schedule without first consulting their physicians. Neither the publisher, the producer, or the authors take any responsibility for any possible consequences from any treatment, action or application of medicine or preparation by any person reading or following the information in this book.

IMPORTANT NOTE: This book was written to [illegible] appropriate health professional regarding all [illegible] [illegible] [illegible] [illegible] [illegible] [illegible] [illegible]. Neither the publisher, the producer, nor the author take any responsibility for any possible consequences from any treatment, action, or application of medicine or preparation to any person reading or following the information in this book.

To my wife, Georgette, whose patience and encouragement knows no bounds, and to my children, Noah and Alexa, for teaching me so many things about children that no one ever taught me in school.

—Max Van Gilder, M.D.

As always, to my loving daughter Caitlin

—Shelagh Ryan Masline

CONTENTS

INTRODUCTION

I'm a pediatrician, so my phone rings a lot. Part of every pediatrician's job is to listen and to teach. I explain how problems occur, why they occur, and tell patients what to do about them.

I have resources on every developmental and behavioral problem. But when it comes to medications, the resources I find are either far too technical for a parent, or they simply repeat the boilerplate information required on the package insert. No information source I have found is understandable, objective, and opinionated.

The book you are holding covers prescription and over-the-counter medications for children in clear, plain English. The organization of the information about a drug prescribed or recommended for your child is designed to enable you to understand clearly what the drug is and how it works. Here you will discover the side effects you often see and the side effects you should worry about, and how the medical community views this drug. (That's the opinion part.)

I have paid great attention to the issue of pediatric dosages. I find that patients experience difficulty in calculating drug dosages by weight, something I have to do every day. It requires practice, even though the process is usually simple math. In this book I have given doses for children at a number of weights. If your child falls between these weights, so should the dose of medication.

But sometimes the process is *not* simple mathematics.

Certain drugs cannot be used in smaller children, and other drugs reach the adult limits before the child reaches adult size. In a few instances, children can and should take more medication than adults. This information is incorporated into the dosage tables.

Opinion is important, too. As a parent, you need to know whether a drug is the best current treatment or one that is limited in its usefulness. All opinion is subjective, but I have tried to make these opinions represent mainstream medical opinion based on as much scientific information as we have.

I do have a point of view, however. I have always been taught that the fewer drugs you use, the better your treatment. I don't think every problem a child faces requires a drug to cure it. I think some drugs for relief of symptoms are overused. I don't think that a cold requires a four- or five-drug treatment regimen. I am sure that the cold will not go away one minute earlier because of the treatment. I am convinced that easing the child's discomfort with acetaminophen (Tylenol, Tempra) or ibuprofen (Advil, Motrin) is often all a child needs, although I frequently add a cough suppressant as well so that a child can sleep or go to school. When I review all the wonderful new antibiotics we have developed, I still find that amoxicillin works just fine for the majority of children's infections.

Lastly, I think that we have lost sight of our goal in treating sick children, which is to make them feel better. Comforting a child with attention, touch, and maybe a little chicken soup will cure 50 percent of the world's problems (perhaps I exaggerate). Let's use important drugs for the real problems, and not try to find a drug to make every little problem go away.

MAX VAN GILDER, M.D.

HOW TO USE THIS BOOK

This book is designed to help parents become well-informed consumers regarding prescription and over-the-counter medications for their children. As a parent, your job is to help your sick child feel better and get well. Yet, with the enormous variety of drugs on the market today, it is not always easy to sort out what is best for your child. In this book you will learn all you need to know about the medications you give your child from birth to age ten.

In Chapter One we discuss how to form a successful partnership with your pediatrician to keep your child healthy. Here we consider the vital importance of effective communication with your child's doctor.

In Chapter Two we look at the easiest ways to administer medications to your child. There are many ways to encourage children—even when they are unwilling or reluctant—to take the medicine that will make them better. We also review the many different types of medications available for children.

In Chapter Three we explore the components of a well-stocked home medicine cabinet and first-aid kit. Here you'll learn how to equip yourself with all the necessities for day-to-day care, as well as items to have on hand in case of medical emergencies.

In Chapter Four we consider immunizations, one of the most valuable tools we have to protect our children from disease. We also examine the antivaccination controversy. Many parents are genuinely concerned that immunizations may pose hidden risks to children.

In Chapter Five you will find an easy-to-use and accessible A-to-Z guide to the medications most frequently prescribed for children. Drugs are alphabetized by their generic name. If you don't know the generic name of a drug you'd like to look up, turn to the index at the back of the book and look up the brand name. In each profile you will find invaluable information about the medication, including: appropriate dosages; how to best administer the medication; possible side effects and adverse reactions; and important precautions. When discussing side effects, we separate those that are common and harmless from those adverse reactions that may require discontinuing the medication and consulting with your pediatrician.

In Chapter Six we turn to over-the-counter medications. Again, the profiles are arranged alphabetically by generic name, and you can use the index at the back of the book to look up familiar brand names. Each profile will include general information about the medication: details about dosage and administration; side effects and adverse reactions to watch out for; and important precautions. Once more, we separate common side effects from more potentially serious adverse reactions.

While no book can replace the care and attention of your pediatrician, becoming knowledgeable about the medications you give your child is one of the most important things you can do to assure their well-being and your peace of mind.

1

USING MEDICATION SAFELY: What You Need to Know

With all the runny noses, sore throats, earaches, and upset stomachs that your child experiences, it may often seem that childhood is just one long list of ailments. Happily, most childhood illnesses are not very serious and children tend to bounce back quickly from them. Even the more serious diseases, such as pneumonia or bacterial meningitis, are rarely life-threatening, and are usually treated successfully with no long-term effects.

Medications can help your child feel better and get well. Both prescription and nonprescription (also known as over-the-counter, or OTC) drugs are safe and effective when used properly, yet each can have serious or even dire side effects if you neglect to follow your pediatrician's instructions or the package directions. With that in mind, here are some basic safety guidelines to follow when giving medications to your child.

A Child Is Not a Miniature Adult

Never give your child medicine that has been prescribed for an adult. Remember that kids are not just small adults. Children metabolize drugs differently than adults, sometimes more slowly, sometimes more rapidly. This means that potentially dangerous levels of drugs can accumulate more quickly in a child than in an adult. A safe and effective drug for Mommy's headache may prove to be a very dangerous remedy indeed for Baby. Special formulations of medications are both necessary and appropriate for children. Sometimes children need entirely different medications than adults.

Always give your child the precise dosage of medication appropriate to his or her age and weight. It's equally important to administer the medicine correctly, following the instructions from your pediatrician or included with the package information.

No manufacturer is allowed to give instructions for children under the age of twenty-four months, so it's best to consult your pediatrician before giving any medication to children under two. (In Chapter Two we'll give detailed information on the administration of medications.)

Side Effects and Adverse Reactions

Before giving *any* prescription medication to your child, be sure to ask your pediatrician if you should anticipate any side effects or adverse reactions. When you choose an over-the-counter product for your child, read the label carefully to obtain this information. Be aware that each child's response to a medication is highly individual; different children from the same family may tolerate medications differently.

Recommended dosages of medication are based on your child's body weight as well as age. Surprisingly, children's doses are sometimes higher than those of adults and can cause fewer side effects.

Immediately discontinue any prescription or nonprescription drug if your child develops a troubling response to it, and contact your pediatrician to see what further action is necessary. If your child develops reactions such as a rash, a loss of balance, or excessive sleepiness, call your pediatrician. In the case of a more serious adverse reaction, such as a convulsion, difficulty breathing, or loss of consciousness, immediate action is required. Take your child to the nearest emergency room for treatment. Bring all medicines the child has taken—or *might* have taken—with you.

Allergic Reactions to Drugs

An allergic reaction can range from a harmless stomachache to cardiac arrest and death. Whenever you give your child a medication for the first time, watch him or her carefully for any unusual symptoms. Also be aware that some children who have taken a medication previously with no complications can develop an allergic reaction out of the blue. This is because the body can become sensitized to an allergen over time.

A very severe and potentially life-threatening allergic reaction is called anaphylaxis. Anaphylaxis is characterized by a sudden onset of hives, difficulty breathing, and extreme pallor caused by a drop in blood pressure that can result in coma or cardiac arrest.

If your child goes into anaphylactic shock, call 911 and describe your child's symptoms. Do not try to take your child to the emergency room yourself unless told to do so by emergency personnel. Tell the 911 operator that you need an ambulance immediately.

Anaphylaxis can be caused by a number of allergens, including penicillin and other antibiotics, insect venom, vaccines, food (such as seafood, nuts, or egg whites), and aspirin.

AVOID ALL PRODUCTS THAT CONTAIN ASPIRIN

Unless specifically directed to do so by your pediatrician, do not give your child aspirin or other medications that contain aspirin. Children who are given these products, particularly when they have chicken pox, flu, or flulike symptoms, may develop a life-threatening condition called Reye syndrome. Children should instead be given acetaminophen, which safely reduces pain and fever. Ibuprofen, which has recently shifted from a prescription to an OTC medication for children, is another safe and helpful treatment alternative not associated with Reye syndrome.

The symptoms of Reye syndrome usually occur toward the end of the original illness, and may include extreme tiredness, violent headache, disorientation, belligerence, and repeated vomiting. Read the label before purchasing *any* OTC medication.

The following products do not have aspirin in their brand names, but contain aspirin (or related compounds called salicylates) and should not be taken by children or teenagers:

- Alka-Seltzer Effervescent Antacid and Pain Reliever
- Alka-Seltzer Plus Night-Time Cold Medicine
- Anacin Maximum Strength Analgesic Coated Tablets
- Ascriptin A/D Caplets
- BC Powder
- BC Cold Powder Multi-Symptom Formula
- BC Cold Powder NonDrowsy Formula
- Bufferin (all formulations)
- Excedrin Extra-Strength Analgesic Tablets and Caplets
- Pepto-Bismol
- Ursinus Inlay-Tabs
- Vanquish Analgesic Tablets

Two Categories of Medicine: Prescription and Over-the-Counter

There are two basic types of medication: prescription and nonprescription (OTC). Prescription drugs require a special prescription from your pediatrician that can only be filled at your pharmacy; over-the-counter medications are available on the shelves of supermarkets and convenience stores as well as pharmacies.

Both prescription and nonprescription drugs contain powerful chemicals that can be harmful if not taken properly. This is why medications of *all* kinds should be stored safely out of the reach of children.

Prescription Drugs

Medicines are generally classified as "available by prescription only" if there is a substantial risk of side effects or adverse reactions, if there is a substantial possibility of interaction with other medications, or if the patient taking the prescription requires close medical supervision during the medication period. Prescription drugs are regulated by the FDA (Food and Drug Administration).

Many childhood ailments—such as middle ear infections, strep throat, or a severe allergic reaction—require a visit to your pediatrician for diagnosis and treatment. If your pediatrician prescribes medication for your child, you should not be alarmed. A prescription drug does not necessarily indicate that the underlying ailment is severe; it may simply mean that an antibiotic is the most appropriate treatment for your child's bacterial infection, or that a prescription drug is available that can halt your child's allergic reaction and ease his or her difficulty in breathing.

BRAND NAME OR GENERIC?

Many prescription drugs are available in two versions: generic and brand. The smart comparison-shopper recognizes that the generic version of most prescription medicines costs much less than the brand name. Yet, while generic drugs are often a good alternative, whether or not they are appropriate for your child should be judged on a case-by-case basis by your pediatrician.

In many situations, the composition, quality, and effectiveness of generic drugs *are* largely equivalent to that of more expensive brand name products. In other cases, generic drugs are less effective than their brand name counterparts. Sometimes the principal drug ingredient in a generic medication may be accompanied by inert additives that may prevent the desired therapeutic effect on your child. Whenever your pediatrician fills out a prescription for your child, make it a habit to ask if the generic drug is a safe and effective alternative to the brand name. If you *want* the brand name product, the prescription must specifically state this.

ASKING THE RIGHT QUESTIONS ABOUT PRESCRIPTION MEDICATIONS

Medical treatment consists of a good partnership between you and your pediatrician, the goal of which is to keep your child healthy. One of the hallmarks of a successful partnership is effective communication. As a parent, your job is to accurately describe your child's symptoms to your pediatrician, advise him or her of any drug allergies your child may have, and report all other medications you are presently giving your child (in case of drug interactions).

Your pediatrician's job is not only to diagnose and treat your child's illness correctly but also to answer your questions. Jot down your questions before going to each medical appointment; questions are often more difficult to recall during the actual examination. When your pediatrician writes a prescription, important questions to ask include:

- What is the proper dosage?
- How often should doses be given?
- What should I do if I forget to give my child a dosage at the proper time?
- Should the drug be taken with or without food?
- Do any foods interfere with the medication's effectiveness?
- Should I administer a new dose of medication immediately if my child spits out or vomits up the first dose?
- Should I interrupt my child's sleep to administer medication?
- What side effects should I watch out for?
- Have there been any dangerous adverse reactions to the drug?
- How soon should I expect to see an improvement?
- Should I discontinue medication if my child appears better?
- Can I keep leftover medication in case of a possible recurrence of the problem?
- Is the prescription renewable?
- Is it safe to give my child OTC medications while he or she is taking this prescription?
- Can I safely use a generic version instead of the brand name prescription?
- When should I contact you again?

Over-the-Counter Medications

Surveys show that nine out of ten Americans attend to everyday aches and pains without consulting a health professional. Sometimes we simply wait until symptoms disappear on their own; other times we use a home remedy; very often we choose an over-the-counter product. Most parents keep a number of over-the-counter supplies on hand in case of emergency. (Turn to Chapter Three for a complete list of the equipment you should keep in your own home medicine cabinet and first-aid kit.)

Consumers who don't seek medical advice are pretty much on their own when using over-the-counter products. Because of this, the FDA requires that OTC labels include a great deal of information. Whenever you purchase an over-the-counter medication for your child, take full advantage of this information, which will include not only proper dosage and administration, but also possible side effects and adverse reactions.

OTC DRUGS ARE SERIOUS MEDICINE

Over-the-counter drugs, while safe and effective when used correctly, are still very serious medicine and should not be given to children in an offhand way. It's easy to get casual about a seemingly innocuous medicine your child has been using for years, but OTC preparations should be handled with care.

More medications are being made available all the time on a nonprescription basis. This is yet another reason it is so important to read labels *carefully* and to follow the instructions written on them *exactly.*

Choosing the Right OTC Medication

When choosing OTC medication for your child, avoid combination products that promise to relieve or cure all your child's ills. These products often do more harm than good by overmedicating children—that is, treating children for symptoms they don't even have and exposing them to unnecessary side effects.

Choose medications specific to the symptoms your child is experiencing. For example, an antihistamine blocks the release of histamine and dries up a runny nose; the purpose of a decongestant is to shrink swollen membranes and thereby unstuff nasal passages.

Be sure to check with your pediatrician before giving

your child different medications to treat different symptoms. Many products contain overlapping ingredients; if you give your child a cough syrup and a cold pill with the same ingredient, an overdose could result.

Most over-the-counter medications are for symptom relief. This means they will not *cure* any underlying illness or disorder. If your child is suffering from an ear infection, for example, acetaminophen may ease the accompanying pain and fever, but it will not clear up the actual infection. If she has bronchitis, cough syrup can soothe her throat and provide relief from coughing, but she may still need a prescription antibiotic.

In most cases, recovery from a disease does not depend on the use of over-the-counter drugs. Many childhood ailments, such as colds, chicken pox, and other viruses, must simply run their course. In a special chart in Chapter Six, we take a closer look at cold and cough remedies, the most commonly used over-the-counter medications for children. OTC medications help you make your child as comfortable as possible while he or she recovers.

If you have any questions about whether or not an over-the-counter medication is appropriate for your child, be sure to speak with your pharmacist or pediatrician.

How to Be a Well-Informed Consumer

In addition to talking to your pediatrician, you obviously will want to read about specific medications in this book. Pharmacists are also excellent sources of information about OTC and prescription medications. Ask your pharmacist if he or she has an information sheet to give you on the drug. Some pharmacies provide printed information with prescription drugs.

Look for the following information on the labels of OTC products or in the printed information that accompanies prescriptions:

- The brand name of the product and the type of drug it is (for example, antibiotic, analgesic, antihistamine)
- A list of the active ingredients (in case your child is allergic to one of the ingredients)
- Warnings (such as whether the drug is appropriate for young children, possible side effects, drug interactions, and when to discontinue use of the product)
- The symptoms the product is intended to treat
- Drug interaction precautions
- Instructions for use (the amount of medicine you should give your child, how often, and method of administering it)
- Information about tamper-evident features (for example, the label may specify that a product is unsafe if a seal is broken)
- The expiration date (the month and year after which the drug will no longer work). Giving your child the drug after this time could be harmful.

THE PROPER DISPOSAL OF MEDICATIONS

Check your medicine cabinet twice a year, and dispose of any prescription medications you no longer take and all OTC medications that have expired. Flush expired drugs down your toilet. *Don't* simply dump them in your garbage, where they may still be accessible. Also dispose of:

- Chipped, cracked, or discolored tablets
- Capsules that have softened and stick together
- Thickened or discolored liquids
- Cracked or leaking tubes
- Discolored, hardened, or separated ointments
- Any tablet, capsule, liquid, ointment, or cream that has an odor different from its original one

Avoiding Accidental Poisoning

Keeping your home safe for your child is the best way to avoid cases of accidental poisoning and other serious emergencies. The greatest number of poisonings in the home occur in the kitchen, followed by the bathroom and bedroom.

Try to make sure that your entire home is completely childproofed—a safe and wholesome environment for your child to grow up in. To avoid accidental poisoning:

- Do not keep poisonous plants in your home, yard, or garden. As many as one percent of all plant species may be toxic to humans. The list of poisonous plants includes belladonna, oleander, poinsettia, hemlock, yew, and wisteria.
- In the kitchen and bathroom, keep all chemical cleansers tightly capped or closed and stored properly—out of the reach of children, preferably in a locked cabinet.
- Store all medicine, vitamins, and minerals in childproof containers.
- Keep all liquor bottles tightly closed. Put them on a high shelf or, preferably, in a locked cabinet.
- In the garage or basement, keep all chemicals (such as pesticides and weed killers) tightly closed.
- Keep paint and paint products tightly closed. Throw out all old paint.
- Thoroughly clean up any oil or gasoline spills.
- Never store toxic substances in drinking containers, including soda bottles or drinking cups.

While parents of children of all ages should take precautions against accidental poisoning, parents of toddlers should pay particular attention to this problem. One way toddlers explore their world is by putting colorful and interesting new discoveries into their mouths. Not surprisingly, the greatest danger of accidental poisoning is in this age group. Infants do not yet have the mobility to get into this type of trouble, and once your child reaches school age you can usually reason with her and explain why certain things are dangerous.

What to Do in a Poisoning Emergency

Any time a child has swallowed or is suspected of having swallowed an inappropriate prescription or nonprescription drug or other substance, emergency action is necessary. Call your poison control center and carefully follow their instructions. Do *not* phone 911. Although the operator always has the poison center number, you'll save precious seconds if the number is posted near your phone. In my practice, I hand out a sticker with the phone number of the local poison control center and tell the parents of my young patients to tape it to the kitchen telephone, as well as program it into their auto-dialer if they have one.

Ipecac and activated charcoal are the two most important items to keep in your home in case of accidental posioning. Depending upon the poison your child has ingested, the poison control operator may instruct you to administer one of these to your child.

If you are directed to an emergency room, be sure to bring any empty bottles, remaining medicine, and/or a specimen of your child's vomit with you for analysis. Effective treatment of accidental poisoning depends on a doctor making a rapid decision based on the nature and amount of a drug taken.

Emergency action is needed and poisoning should be suspected if your child develops one or more of the following symptoms:

- Extreme drowsiness or loss of consciousness
- Shallow or irregular breathing
- Repeated vomiting
- Convulsions

When children are sick, the two goals of concerned parents and pediatricians are to help them get well quickly and, in the meantime, to ease their discomfort. As you have seen in this chapter, medications—when used correctly and responsibly—can help you achieve these joint goals. In the chapter that follows, you will learn more about the safe and effective administration of medications.

2

HOW TO GIVE MEDICINE TO YOUR CHILD

Getting a child to take medicine is not always an easy task. Children may be too young to understand the benefits of medicine, or too tired and ill to care. Some children refuse to take medicine simply to challenge Mom, while others reject it on the basis of taste. If a medicine is particularly unpalatable, it may be necessary to contact your pediatrician for advice, or a new prescription. Fortunately, however, there are many tried-and-true techniques that can help you coax your reluctant child to take her medicine.

Coaxing the Reluctant Child

How you get children to take medicine often depends on their age and personality. A generally compliant child may offer no resistance, while a rebellious two-year-old may reject medicine in much the same manner that she routinely says "no" to everything else. Following are a few techniques that may help your child cooperate.

Be Firm Yet Gentle

A firm but light touch meets with the greatest success when administering medicine to children. You must try to remain calm—and try to keep your child calm as well—even as you gently insist that she follow a course of action that doesn't hold much appeal. As soon as your child has even a tiny understanding of cause and effect, you can try to explain that you are giving her the medicine because she is feeling sick now, and after she takes the medicine she will feel better. After giving medicine to your child, hold or gently rock her, and calm her with the familiar and soothing tone of your voice.

Honesty Is the Best Policy

Just as you shouldn't pretend that the shot they get at the doctor's office isn't going to hurt, it's best to prepare children when medicine has a bitter taste. Honesty is truly the best policy. If you mislead your child even once to get the medicine down, you are creating a new reservoir of stubborn resistance to all future attempts.

KEEP YOUR COOL

Try to be matter-of-fact about the whole business. Don't raise your voice or make idle threats. Children quickly pick up on any tension that you yourself may be feeling, and tension and anxiety will only worsen the situation.

ROLE-PLAYING AND PLAYACTING

Unless you have significant allergies, it's not a bad idea to taste test the medicine yourself. Your child will see that you've taken it—and you've survived. Perhaps you can pretend to give some to the child's favorite dolls and stuffed animals as well. And if you make a funny face, your child may even get into the spirit of playacting with you. Afterward, if the medicine is bitter, you can all share a plate of plain crackers to take away the taste.

POSITIVE REINFORCEMENT

Some parents are initially put off by this strategy, thinking of rewards for cooperation as consisting solely of sugary lollipops or other sweets. Yet positive reinforcement of a child's cooperation might also consist of nonsugar alternatives, such as a chart with stars on it: one star for each dosage of medication, and, possibly, one for every time you take your child's temperature. The completed chart of stars may be reward enough for many children; or, upon completion, you might let your child choose a simple, inexpensive present, such as a new coloring book and crayons.

MEDICINE IS NOT CANDY

While you may literally be willing to stand on your head to get your child to take her medicine, never make the mistake of portraying medicine as candy. Scrupulous as you may be about storing your medicine, if you slip up once and leave medicine lying around—or if your child comes upon medicine at the home of a friend or relative—your child may think it is candy and eat it, and you may have a frightening case of accidental poisoning on your hands.

Safe and Effective Administration of Medicine

Medications come in many shapes and forms, such as liquids, tablets, capsules, drops, creams, ointments, sprays, and inhalers. The majority of medications are administered orally; some are more effective when taken on an empty stomach, while others should be taken with meals. In many cases, such as a course of antibiotics, it's important for your child to continue to take medication even after symptoms have disappeared. Ask your pediatrician or pharmacist for instructions, and don't forget to carefully read all labels.

Following are guidelines to the safe and effective administration of a variety of medications frequently recommended or prescribed for children.

LIQUID PREPARATIONS

Liquid preparations are the most common form of medicine for young children. You can give your child a liquid medication using a dropper, oral syringe, spoon, or medicine cup. An infant may be given medicine in a nipple. Do not use a regular household spoon to administer medicine to your child, since this is not a sufficiently exact measurement. Over time, see what method your child is most comfortable with. Medicine droppers and nipples are often easiest and most appropriate for infants, while toddlers can graduate to calibrated spoons or cups.

To administer liquid medicine to infants, place a little of the liquid at a time into the side or back corner of the baby's mouth. (Never aim medicine toward the center of a baby's mouth; this can cause gagging or choking.) If the baby rejects the medicine and spits it out—a common reaction, and one all too familiar to most parents—simply persevere. Put a little more medicine in her cheek, and this time gently but firmly close your baby's mouth until she swallows it.

Administering liquid medicines to toddlers and preschoolers is usually easier. If you use a spoon, try to put the liquid on the back of your child's tongue for fastest and most efficient swallowing. At this age, most children can also manage a cup. (Most liquid cold preparations come with their own calibrated plastic cups on top.) Have a favorite drink or cracker ready to wash away any medicinal aftertaste.

Liquid preparations for children come in three forms:

- *Elixir*—Elixirs have traditionally been defined as clear mixtures of the active ingredients of a drug combined with flavored alcohol. However, many of the elixirs available today do not contain alcohol.
- *Suspension*—Suspensions are cloudy mixtures in which active ingredients are mixed with flavoring agents. Suspensions must be shaken well, since active ingredients may settle to the bottom of the bottle.
- *Syrup*—Clear syrups are mixtures of the active ingredients of a drug with sugar-based flavoring agents.

TABLETS

While liquid medicine is the appropriate method of delivering most drugs to infants, you have more options with older children. Tablets can be crushed between two spoons and the resulting powder mixed with your child's favorite food: for example, cereal, applesauce, or ice cream. Many toddlers and preschoolers are willing to take fruit-flavored chewable tablets. (Take care that you watch your child take the medication; no tablets or other drugs should be left in the reach of children.)

CAPSULES

Solid gelatin-coated tablets may be easier for your child to swallow than pills. Wetting them makes these capsules even easier to swallow. Enteric-coated capsules are often recommended for intestinal disorders, since they do not dissolve and release their active ingredients until they reach the intestinal area past the stomach; therefore it would be defeating their purpose to administer them by breaking and mixing their contents with food or drink. Speak to your pediatrician if you are having problems administering enteric-coated capsules to your child.

EYEDROPS AND OINTMENT

Eyedrops and ointment are often prescribed to treat a common childhood ailment known as conjunctivitis, or pinkeye. Conjunctivitis, an inflammation of the eye, is extremely contagious. An eyedropper, which comes with the prescribed solution, is easily infected and should never be shared. The eyedrops should be administered at room temperature. If your pediatrician recommends treating both your child's eyes, even if only one eye is infected so far, be sure to treat the uninfected eye first. Also be certain not to touch the tip of the eyedropper, for fear of contamination. It is not necessary to sterilize the dropper after each treatment. If contamination occurs, however, discard the medicine.

Do not expect much cooperation from your child when it comes to giving eyedrops. The best-intentioned child is still subject to her own reflexes; that is, when a dropper is coming at her eye, she blinks. Hold your child in your lap with her head back, and gently use your finger and thumb to hold eyelids apart; then drop the solution into the inner corner of the eye. You may have to do this several times before you are sure some solution has actually entered the eye. Two people can often manage this process better than one.

The application of eye ointment is often easier and more pleasant for your child. Eye ointments come in small tubes with tiny nozzles on the end. Simply squeeze the correct amount into the inner corner of the eye. Hold your child still so that the ointment can spread across the eye, making sure she doesn't simply wipe it away.

EARDROPS

Medicine for middle ear infections, one of the most common childhood ailments, must be given orally. But eardrops are often prescribed for local outer ear infections, such as swimmer's ear. Before administering eardrops, warm the bottle of solution slightly by holding under a stream of hot water; then test a few drops on your inner wrist to make sure they are not too hot.

Next, lie your child sideways across your lap and administer the correct number of drops into the ear. Aim at the wall of the ear canal. Keep your child still for a minute or two, so eardrops do not drain out. Never share eardroppers or ear medication, and be sure not to touch the tip of the eardropper, which may be contaminated. Any contaminated medicine should be discarded.

NOSE DROPS

Nose drops, like eyedrops, should be administered at room temperature. Your pediatrician may prescribe nose drops for infants whose nasal passages are blocked. Nose drops should be used only when recommended by your doctor. They should not be shared or reused, since nose droppers can spread infection.

Before administering nose drops, you may want to use a bulb syringe, called a nasal aspirator, to remove some of the mucus. Then tilt your baby's head back gently against a pillow (remember at all times to continue to support the head), and squeeze the recommended number of drops into each nostril. Be careful not to insert the dropper all the way into either nostril, which can cause possible injury or contamination.

SHAMPOO

Medicated shampoo is generally indicated for allergic scalp conditions such as seborrhea. More specialized shampoos are also available to rid your child of uncomfortable and highly contagious infestations of head lice or scabies. Be extremely careful not to allow medicated shampoo, which contains irritating chemical ingredients, to get into your child's eyes.

Following the instructions on the label of the medicated

shampoo, carefully wash your child's hair. When possible, use a portable shower head to contain shampoo to the scalp area, and protect your child's eyes by covering them with a towel. After shampooing, rinse the hair very thoroughly.

SKIN MEDICATIONS

Ointments and other topical medications are ordinarily very easy to apply. Wash your own hands with soap and water, and apply the medication evenly over your child's skin. Children are usually willing to cooperate, since skin medications are formulated to provide relief of their rash, sting, bite, itch, wound, or cut. Children should be reminded, of course, that these medications do not go in or near their mouths and eyes.

Skin medications come in all varieties: ointment, lotion, gel, etcetera. It is best to adhere to the recommended dosages. More ointment does not necessarily mean more curing power.

Most cuts and scrapes can be handled with soap and water and an adhesive bandage strip. (OTC antibiotic ointments and creams have never been proven effective in preventing infection, although many parents feel a greater sense of security once they are applied to a child's wound.) Rashes in infants under three months should be treated only by your pediatrician. For older children, over-the-counter medications, oatmeal baths, and short fingernails are effective rash care. For more serious wounds, apply a pressure bandage to stop bleeding and seek emergency treatment.

SUPPOSITORIES

Suppositories are small, bullet-shaped tablets containing a mixture of drugs with glycerin. They are inserted into a child's rectum, where they melt and allow the drug to be absorbed. Suppositories are usually prescribed when very young children are nauseous and unable to keep down oral medications. They should not be given unless specifically recommended by your pediatrician, and should be used with care.

To insert a suppository, have your child lay on his side with her knees pulled up to her chest. Hold the suppository with a piece of toilet paper or paper towel. Put Vaseline™ on the suppository for easier insertion, spread your child's buttocks, and gently insert the suppository completely into the rectum. Hold the buttocks together for a moment, so the suppository is lodged and begins to dissolve.

A Checklist: Safety Tips for Giving Medicine to Children

- Never give aspirin to any child under the age of eighteen. Aspirin has been linked with Reye syndrome, a rare but serious condition that may affect a child's brain and liver.
- Never give your child a drug to which she has previously experienced a sensitive reaction, such as a rash, swollen joints, nausea, diarrhea, or vomiting.
- Keep all medication out of the reach of children.
- Never give your child a medication that was prescribed for an adult or for another child.
- Make sure your pharmacist puts all prescription drugs in childproof containers.
- Do not use any medication that is opened or shows other signs of tampering.
- In the case of prescription medicine, complete the entire course of medication prescribed by your pediatrician, even if your child's symptoms disappear. Failure to do so may prevent your child's complete recovery.
- Carefully read and follow the instructions on over-the-counter medications.
- Do not give your child over-the-counter medications

for long periods of time without consulting your pediatrician.

- Do not exceed the recommended dosage for *any* medication without specific recommendations from your pediatrician.
- Do not dilute your child's medicine unless specifically instructed to do so by your pediatrician.
- Do not add medicine to your baby's bottle.
- Check expiration dates. Replace over-the-counter medications on a yearly basis.
- Store all drugs in a locked medicine cabinet.
- Store medications at room temperature. Avoid high humidity and excessive heat.
- If you have questions or concerns about any medication, ask your pediatrician or pharmacist for advice.
- Do not give your child more than the indicated amount of medication in any 24-hour period. Severe or recurring pain may be a sign of serious illness. Under these conditions, consult your pediatrician.
- In case of accidental overdosage, contact your physician or poison control center immediately.

GIVING MEDICINE TO CHILDREN: THE KEYS TO SUCCESS

In order to successfully give medicine to your child:

- Be firm, yet also gentle; try to keep your child calm.
- Be honest about the taste of the medicine.
- Try to be patient with your child.
- Use role-playing and playacting to lessen your child's anxiety about taking medicine.
- Offer your child positive reinforcement for successfully coping with the experience.

3

FIRST AID IN THE HOME

There's no way around it: your child is going to collect any number of cuts, scrapes, and bruises on the bumpy road to adulthood. But with the help of a well-stocked home medicine cabinet, you'll be able to handle day-to-day mishaps with hugs, kisses, and a good supply of Band-Aids™, antiseptic, and common sense.

A home first-aid kit is also recommended by most medical experts. This is a collection of articles designed to handle more serious medical emergencies. Hopefully you'll never have to use it—but you can rest easier knowing that you have the ipecac and emergency numbers on hand, just in case. In the meantime, remember that prevention is always the best remedy.

Your Home Medicine Cabinet

You will find that only a small number of items is actually needed to deal with a whole multitude of common childhood problems, such as cuts and scrapes, colds, fever, and flu. The truth is, you simply don't have time to run out to the store when your baby wakes in the middle of the night with a fever, or when your preschooler takes a spill on his bike. It's best to keep essential supplies in your own medicine cabinet to cope with the situation at hand. Acetaminophen, for example, will relieve a fever, while soap and water, a Band-Aid, and a hug are the standard cure for a scrape.

Your home medicine cabinet is the best place to store your collection of standard medical supplies. Remember, prescription and over-the-counter drugs should be kept in a locked medicine cabinet or on a high closet shelf, safely out of the reach of children. Medications should also be kept in a dry and cool environment to retain their potency.

Some basic items to include in your home medicine cabinet are:

ACETAMINOPHEN

Acetaminophen relieves mild pain and fever in children, making it an indispensable part of every family's medicine cabinet. Acetaminophen is an analgesic—that is, a pain and fever reliever—and is available in generic form, as well as under brand names, such as Tylenol and Tempra.

Acetaminophen is by far the safest over-the-counter analgesic. Keep in mind that aspirin, probably the analgesic most commonly used by adults, is rarely appropriate for children, and should only be used when specifically recommended by your pediatrician. Aspirin has been linked with a rare yet potentially fatal disease known as Reye syndrome, especially when administered to relieve flulike symptoms in children of eighteen and younger.

ADHESIVE BANDAGES

Adhesive bandages, or Band-Aids, are a normal part of growing up. Manufacturers are well aware of this fact, and pharmacy shelves are jam-packed with neon Band-Aids that glow in the dark and Band-Aids featuring your child's favorite cartoon characters. Let your toddler choose their favorite Band-Aid, and you will have already taken a little of the sting out of the next boo-boo.

A MILD SOAP

Proper removal of contamination with simple soap and water is the most effective means of preventing infection when cleaning a cut or scrape. Choose a mild, unscented soap. Studies show that special antibacterial soaps do little to prevent infection of cuts and scrapes (although they are helpful in preventing the passage of bacteria from one surface to another by way of the hands).

ANTIBACTERIAL/ANTIBIOTIC OINTMENT

Studies show that antibacterial or antibiotic ointments, such as Neosporin and Bacitracin, do little to prevent infection of cuts and scrapes—but many parents feel that they can be soothing and comforting to a child (and to themselves). If foreign bodies (dirt, pebbles, etcetera) are left in a wound, no topical antibiotic will prevent infection. If the contaminants are promptly removed the chance of infection is small, and there is little need for an antibacterial or antibiotic ointment. Nonetheless, if it gives you an added sense of security, apply a thin layer of ointment to your child's cut or scrape after washing the affected area.

ANTIHISTAMINES

Oral antihistamines, contrary to popular belief, won't do much for your child's cold—but they *are* a powerful weapon against allergies and allergic reactions to insect bites, stings, and poison ivy. In these cases, antihistamines block the body's release of histamine, a chemical produced in response to allergenic chemicals or inflammation. Histamine can cause fluids to flow into your child's eyes, nose, and sinuses, or cause his skin to become itchy and red.

ANTISEPTICS

Antiseptics are helpful in cleaning wounds and preventing infection. Hydrogen peroxide is probably the most widely used antiseptic. It's inexpensive and effective. The fizzing action cleans the cut and reduces the chances of infection.

PENLIGHT

A small penlight or flashlight is helpful when your child appears to have a sore throat. Severe redness or white spots coating the throat mean you should give your pediatrician a call. Remember to replace batteries on a regular basis; a light with a weak battery will make your child's throat appear red when it is not.

PETROLEUM JELLY

This multipurpose skin protector can ease the discomfort of diaper rash, as well as protect your child's lips, nose, and other sensitive, exposed areas of skin on cold and windy days. If you use a rectal thermometer, a dab of petroleum will lubricate the tip and help make insertion easier and gentler.

RUBBING ALCOHOL

Rubbing alcohol is useful for cleaning thermometers and tweezers after each use. Follow up with a rinse in cold water.

SUNSCREEN

Damage from exposure to the sun is cumulative—that is, it builds up over a lifetime—so you should start now to limit your child's sun exposure. After a baby is six months old, you can apply sunscreen. Choose one with a sun protection factor (SPF) of at least 15 whenever you go outside with your child—whether you're going to the beach or spending the afternoon in the park, and even if it's not a particularly sunny day. An SPF of 15 means that your child can be exposed to the sun 15 times longer than the time period in which his skin would ordinarily begin to burn.

Fair-skinned children are especially susceptible to the harmful effects of the sun. For these children you may want to get a special children's lotion or cream with an SPF of 25 or 30. PABA-free sunscreens are best, since many children have proven to be allergic to PABA. Sunscreens should also be waterproof, since ordinary sunscreens are likely to come off with water or sweating.

Always apply sunscreen liberally, and try to do so at least 15 to 30 minutes before going out. This gives the active ingredients time to sink in and offer effective sun protection. Reapply frequently, and don't neglect vulnerable areas such as your child's lips, nose, and ears.

THERMOMETERS

Taking your child's temperature when he is ill is important. Rectal thermometers, which have thicker and blunter bulbs than oral thermometers, are the best means to measure the body temperatures of children under five. Never use forehead thermometer strips, which can easily give false readings.

To use a rectal thermometer, lay your child stomach-down on your lap with her legs dangling off the side. Gently spread the buttocks to locate the rectal opening, put a little petroleum jelly on the bulb, and carefully insert about one inch into the rectum. Hold in place for three minutes.

Low-grade fevers often resolve themselves without any action on your part. For fevers over 101 degrees Fahrenheit, acetaminophen is the first line of defense. Ibuprofen (Motrin, Advil) has recently become an over-the-counter medication and can be used if acetaminophen is not giving adequate relief of symptoms. As always, check the label and make sure you give the dosage appropriate to your child's age and weight. In the meantime, keep your child cool. Avoid any tendency to overdress him, and try giving him a cool and soothing bath. Children should also be given extra fluids to prevent dehydration.

Continue to use a thermometer to monitor any fever over 100 degrees Fahrenheit. Fevers of 104 degrees Fahrenheit or higher are a cause for concern. Contact your pediatrician if your child's temperature persists, continues to rise, or does not respond to acetaminophen.

YOUR HOME FIRST-AID KIT

A fully stocked first-aid kit will enable you or your caretaker to handle most minor accidents at home. In the case of a more serious medical emergency, call 911 (or your pediatrician or poison control center) and get your child to a doctor immediately. Animal bites, burns, deep lacerations, possible fractures, and head injuries can all constitute emergencies. Take any interim emergency measures recommended by your 911 operator, pediatrician, or poison control center: for example, you may be asked to apply pressure with sterile gauze to stop a wound from bleeding, or to keep a child as calm and still as possible until help arrives.

Your first-aid kit should be kept accessible to you, yet well out of the reach of children. A clearly labeled plastic or metal box is best for storage. Like your medicine cabinet, the first-aid kit should be kept on a shelf in a cool, dry place.

If your child spends time with a babysitter or nanny, it's essential that the caretaker know where you keep your first-aid box, how to open it, and how to use its contents in an emergency situation.

Some basic items to have on hand are:

ADHESIVE BANDAGES

A box of adhesive bandages in an assortment of sizes should be part of your first-aid kit, as well as your medicine cabinet. The ouchless variety is a good idea, for easy removal.

ADHESIVE TAPE

Adhesive tape is necessary to keep sterile gauze pads in place in the case of larger and more serious wounds.

GAUZE BANDAGES AND PADS

Sterile gauze bandages and pads are not as convenient as adhesive pads, since gauze requires adhesive tape to stick to your child's skin. However, gauze bandages and pads provide protection for fresh burns and wounds while allowing them to breathe and begin to heal. They may also be used as pressure bandages to stop bleeding. Include a selection of shapes and sizes in your first-aid kit.

IPECAC AND ACTIVATED CHARCOAL

Always call your poison control center before taking any action with a child you believe has ingested a poison. Syrup of ipecac induces vomiting. But vomiting will only cause further damage, such as throat and stomach injuries, if your child has ingested a corrosive substance (for example, paint thinner, lye, or gasoline). On the other hand, syrup of ipecac or activated charcoal may prove extremely helpful when your child has swallowed an overdose of an OTC medication. But the rule always is: CALL FIRST.

NONSTICK BANDAGES

Telfa or nonstick bandages can be applied over minor wounds and blisters to protect them from friction.

SCISSORS

Include a scissors to cut adhesive tape and gauze pads as necessary.

TWEEZERS

Two types of tweezers should be stored in your first-aid kit: flat-edged and sharply pointed. Flat-edged tweezers are the ideal tool for removing large splinters, while sharply pointed tweezers are better for tiny splinters.

Tweezers should close well, in order to get a good hold on the splinter. Disinfect the tweezers before and after each use with rubbing alcohol, followed by a rinse in cold water.

One caution: Do not use tweezers to remove stingers. The stinger could break off under the skin and lead to further infection. Try a straight-edged object, such as a credit card or the blunt edge of a knife laid flat against the skin, to scrape off and remove a stinger.

EMERGENCY PHONE NUMBERS

A list of emergency phone numbers should be prominently posted by your phone. Also keep a backup list in your first-aid kit:

- 911
- Your pediatrician
- Poison control center

- Police
- Fire department
- Your regular work number
- The number of an emergency contact, such as a trustworthy family member or friend, who you can count on to comfort your child and make any necessary treatment decisions in your absence

A FIRST-AID GUIDE

A book or pamphlet on how to handle common medical emergencies is a helpful addition to every first-aid kit. Remember that it is not always easy to think clearly and act quickly and efficiently in the heat of the moment. The American Academy of Pediatrics' *Caring for Your Baby and Young Child* and *A Sigh of Relief* are two helpful sources to have on hand in emergencies.

In this chapter you have learned about the proper tools to have on hand to cope with day-to-day mishaps and emergencies around the home. You can also take precautions to prevent children from the risk of serious disease. Following a regular course of immunizations, which we outline in Chapter Four, can protect your child from nine very dangerous and possibly even life-threatening afflictions.

4

ALL ABOUT IMMUNIZATIONS

Buckling your baby into a car seat, putting a bicycle helmet on your young rider, childproofing your home—as parents, these are all normal precautions we take to safeguard our children's health. Immunizations are one more valuable tool we have to protect our youngsters from harm.

The era of immunization began in rural nineteenth-century England, when Edward Jenner discovered that milkmaids did not get smallpox. Upon further exploration, he found that it was routine exposure to the cowpox virus that somehow made these workers immune to smallpox.

The groundwork laid by Jenner set the stage for the development of vaccinations that have eradicated some of the deadliest scourges of the twentieth century. Today we have the ability to immunize children against ten diseases: diphtheria, tetanus, pertussis (whooping cough), measles, mumps, rubella (German measles), polio, hemophilus influenza type B (HIB), hepatitis B, and varicella (chicken

Recommended Childhood Immunization Schedule
United States, January - December 1997

Vaccines[1] are listed under the routinely recommended ages. Bars indicate range of acceptable ages for vaccination. Black bars indicate *catch-up vaccination:* at 11-12 years of age, hepatitis B vaccine should be administered to children not previously vaccinated, and Varicella vaccine should be administered to children not previously vaccinated who lack a reliable

Age ▶ / Vaccine ▼	Birth	1 mo	2 mos	4 mos	6 mos	12 mos	15 mos	18 mos	4-6 yrs	11-12 yrs	14-16 yrs
Hepatitis B[2,3]	Hep B-1										
		Hep B-2			Hep B-3					Hep B[3]	
Diphtheria, Tetanus, Pertussis[4]			DTaP or DTP	DTaP or DTP	DTaP or DTP		DTaP or DTP[4]		DTaP or DTP	Td	
H. influenzae type b[5]			Hib	Hib	Hib[5]	Hib[5]					
Polio[6]			Polio[6]	Polio			Polio[6]		Polio		
Measles, Mumps, Rubella[7]						MMR			MMR[7] or	MMR[7]	
Varicella[8]							Var			Var[8]	

Approved by the Advisory Committee on Immunization Practices (ACIP), the American Academy of Pediatrics (AAP), and the American Academy of Family Physicians (AAFP)

1. This schedule indicates the recommended age for routine administration of currently licensed childhood vaccines. Some combination vaccines are available and may be used whenever administration of all components of the vaccine is indicated. Providers should consult the manufacturers' package inserts for detailed recommendations.
2. **Infants born to HBsAg-negative mothers** should receive 2.5mg of Merck vaccine (Recombivax HB) or 10 mg of SmithKline Beecham (SB) vaccine (Engerix-B). The 2nd dose should be administered ⩾ 1 mo after the 1st dose.
   Infants born to HBsAg-positive mothers should receive 0.5 mL hepatitis B immune globulin (HBIG) within 12 hrs of birth, and either 5 μg of Merck vaccine (Recombivax HB) or 10 μg of SB vaccine (Engerix-B) at a separate site. The 2nd dose is recommended at 1-2 mos of age and the 3rd dose at 6 mos of age.
   Infants born to mothers whose HBsAg status is unknown should receive either 5 μg of Merck vaccine (Recombivax HB) or 10 μg of SB vaccine (Engerix-B) within 12 hrs of birth. The 2nd dose of vaccine is recommended at 1 mo of age and the 3rd dose at 6 mos of age. Blood should be drawn at the time of delivery to determine the mother's HBsAg status; if it is positive, the infant should receive HBIG as soon as possible (no later than 1 wk of age). The dosage and timing of subsequent vaccine doses should be based upon the mother's HBsAg status.
3. Children and adolescents who have not been vaccinated against hepatitis B in infancy may begin the series during any childhood visit. Those who have not previously received 3 doses of hepatitis B vaccine should initiate or complete the series during the 11-12 year-old visit. The 2nd dose should be administered at least 1 mo after the 1st dose, and the 3rd dose should be administered at least 4 mos after the 1st dose and at least 2 mos after the 2nd dose.
4. DTaP (diphtheria and tetanus toxoids and acellular pertussis vaccine) is the preferred vaccine for all doses in the vaccination series, including completion of the series in children who have received ⩾ 1 dose of whole-cell DTP vaccine. Whole-cell DTP is an acceptable alternative to DTaP. The 4th dose of DTaP) may be administered as early as 12 months of age, provided 6 months have elapsed since the 3rd dose, and if the child is considered unlikely to return at 15-18 mos of age. Td (tetanus and diphtheria toxoids, absorbed, for adult use) is recommended at 11-12 years of age if at least 5 years have elapsed since the last dose of DTP, DTaP, or DT. Subsequent routine Td boosters are recommended every 10 years.
5. Three *H. influenzae* type b (Hib) conjugate vaccines are licensed for infant use. If PRPOMP (PedvaxHIB [Merck]) is administered at 2 and 4 mos of age, a dose at 6 mos is not required. After completing the primary series, any Hib conjugate vaccine may be used as a booster.
6. Two poliovirus vaccines are currently licensed in the US: inactivated poliovirus vaccine (IPV) and oral poliovirus vaccine (OPV). The following schedules are all acceptable by the ACIP, the AAP, and the AAFP, and parents and providers may choose among them:
   1. IPV at 2 and 4 mos; OPV at 12-18 mos and 4-6 yr
   2. IPV at 2, 4, 12-18 mos, and 4-6 yr
   3. OPV at 2, 4, 6-18 mos, and 4-6 yr

   The ACIP routinely recommends schedule 1. IPV is the only poliovirus vaccine recommended for immunocompromised persons and their household contacts.
7. The 2nd dose of MMR is routinely recommended at 4-6 yrs of age or at 11-12 yrs of age, but may be administered during any visit, provided at least 1 month has elapsed since receipt of the 1st dose and that both doses are administered at or after 12 months of age.
8. Susceptible children may receive Varicella vaccine (Var) at any visit after the first birthday, and those who lack a reliable history of chickenpox should be immunized during the 11-12 year-old visit. Children ⩾ 13 years of age should receive 2 doses, at least 1 mos apart.

pox). All of these diseases, with the exception of tetanus, are contagious, and can lead to disability or even death. We vaccinate against each disease with specific vaccines.

How Vaccines Work

Our bodies have immune cells that are constantly on the lookout for alien substances, with specific cells programmed to seek out and destroy specific invaders. If these invaders break through the body's natural defenses, they are identified and cells are activated to fight them off, most typically by producing antibodies. These antibodies roam the body and, if they come upon the known invader, activate the immune system to isolate, attack, and eliminate the foreign substance.

Vaccines work by helping our bodies produce antibodies to fight off deadly diseases. There are two types of vaccines: live and killed.

LIVE VACCINES

Live vaccines, such as for measles, mumps, and rubella, work by infecting the person with a virus that has been weakened by repeatedly growing it in the laboratory until the virus has evolved into a less potent or less virulent form. Vaccines made in this way cause infection but not disease, and have few side effects.

The infections generated by live vaccines cause the body to produce antibodies, which provide effective protection from the major disease. These vaccines give your child a very, very mild version of the disease—one you probably won't even notice.

KILLED VACCINES

The vaccines for diphtheria, whooping cough, tetanus, HIB, and hepatitis B are made from whole bacteria that have been killed or, in the more recent vaccines, only the parts of the virus or bacteria that cause the body to produce protective antibodies. This approach (unlike that of live vaccines) does not mimic the natural disease process, yet successfully triggers the immune system.

The Immunization Schedule

Many times parents ask whether it would be better to give immunizations separately so as not to overtax a child's immune system. Yet, as we discussed earlier, each disease has a series of cells that produce the specific antibodies for that particular disease. As a result, there is a separate response to each immunization. When we give diphtheria, whooping cough, tetanus, HIB, hepatitis B, and polio immunizations at the same time, each immunization triggers a different group of immune cells. All work independently.

Why Do We Want Every Child Immunized?

Immunizations against diseases are approximately 90 percent effective. That means that if we immunize one hundred children, ninety will make antibodies and be protected. For some reason, not all children respond to an individual immunization. However, if 90 percent of the people your child comes into contact with are protected, then he is far less likely to encounter anyone with an active infection. Likewise, once the level of protection reaches a certain level, the disease cannot spread and dies out.

In some cases, such as whooping cough, the vaccine is only about 45 to 86 percent effective. As a result, whooping cough still exists in the community. In another case, measles, the disease is so contagious that 90 percent immunity is not enough; in recent years, a second MMR (measles, mumps, rubella) vaccination was added to the immunization schedule to raise immunity significantly above the level that is required to halt the spread of the disease. This has been very effective.

The Antivaccination Controversy

Despite the clear benefits of immunization to individual children and to others in the community, many parents today are concerned that immunization poses hidden risks to children. Today, our collective memory of horrifying epidemics has faded, at the same time that health-conscious consumers are far more likely to take an active role in their own medical care. The end result has been a growing anxiety about and distrust of all standard medical treatments—including vaccinations. In the 1980s the media began to broadcast exposés on the evils of the whooping cough (pertussis) vaccine, alleging that these vaccines did more harm than good, and that physicians had been hiding information from the public. To a certain extent, this was true. Physicians have always known that the pertussis vaccine is a problematic vaccine (for detailed information, see page 51). However, it was firmly believed that side effects were a small price to pay for the control of epidemic pertussis. It remains true that a sore arm or slight fever are still the most common side effects of immunization.

Nonetheless, horror stories and accusations of injury resulting from the pertussis vaccine were quickly followed by lawsuits against physicians and manufacturers. The cost of the DPT (diphtheria, tetanus, pertussis) vaccine increased by 1500 percent. A movement against all vaccinations arose, with protesters consisting of groups of parents with ill children, back-to-basics groups, and individuals who felt that many vaccine companies were profiteering. Scientific studies and facts were thrown about without critical evaluation of the data. Individual experiences, pop psychology, and science were all mixed together in a witch's brew, to which the medical establishment made an anemic and ineffective reply.

SEPARATING MYTH FROM REALITY

As you make decisions about vaccinations for your own child, it's important to separate the myths and selective science advanced by antivaccination groups—however well-intended—from the hard facts about the immunization process:

Myth: Improving health and sanitation standards of society caused the major improvements in health, and serious diseases would have disappeared without immunizations.

Fact: It is quite true that improving nutrition, public health, and sanitation have greatly improved the well-being of society as a whole—but they have not necessarily had an impact on the diseases we discuss here.

In many cases, such as measles, the fatality rate has decreased, but the incidence has not. In the case of polio, improved living standards reduced infant exposure to disease. As a result, polio struck later, at an age when it was more likely to cause paralysis. In other cases, such as tetanus, living standards are irrelevant, since tetanus is a germ found in soil. Tetanus exposure results from the accidental contact of soil with open wounds. In the case of hepatitis B, social issues—such as drug use and unprotected promiscuity—are at work, and relate poorly to society's living standards.

Myth: Immunizations are not as good as natural immunity.

Fact: Scientific evidence demonstrates that most immunizations produce the same type and intensity of immunity as the natural disease. Yet there are exceptions in both directions. Diphtheria disease does not produce a lasting immunity, and natural disease is in fact *less* effective than the vaccine. The rubella vaccine, on the other hand, produces a lower level of immunity than the natural disease—yet it is still adequate. The immunity transmitted to babies for rubella, which protects them for the first year of life, may be inadequate, and continues to be the subject of research.

Myth: Immunizations cause autoimmune disease.
Fact: Autoimmune diseases are diseases in which the body attacks itself. There is no evidence in scientific literature to support this assertion, which is pure speculation. People making this argument state that no autoimmune diseases were known before immunizations began. This is not true. Most autoimmune diseases were recognized before widespread immunizations began and, moreover, diseases exist before scientists discover them. There is no belief in the scientific community that autoimmune diseases are new—only newly recognized.

Both bacteria and viruses have been implicated in autoimmune diseases. Some autoimmune diseases appear to require both a genetic predisposition *and* an infection with a bacteria or virus. At this time, only wild or "natural" bacteria and viruses have been implicated. The one possible exception to this is arthritis in adult women who are vaccinated against rubella. (See the section on rubella, page 45.)

THE IMPORTANCE OF READING CRITICALLY

Physicians are scientists, at least part of the time. The scientific method requires an objective study of a problem with comparisons to people who are not affected. These are called controlled studies. Controlled studies on white laboratory rats are easy. Controlled studies on homogeneous populations, such as the Japanese or the Finns, are relatively easy. Studies on the heterogeneous population of the United States are extremely difficult.

The old saying, "There are lies, damn lies, and statistics" applies to any discussion of vaccines. There are good studies and bad studies, and one can quote statistics to buttress any viewpoint. If you read any of the antivaccination articles, beware of comments like these:

Look what happened to my child.

Nothing is more compelling than a picture of a severely disabled child. A picture of a child in a wheelchair decorates many antivaccination articles, and makes for good television. However, what makes a great visual example is not good science. The more carefully done studies in the United States and Great Britain have failed to demonstrate injury from the pertussis vaccine, despite the great hue and cry. Unfortunately, serious illness does occasionally occur in small children—but it is very rarely due to the vaccines we use.

Even the United States government gave up on the smallpox vaccine in 1970.

This is true—but the reason the government recommended that the smallpox vaccine no longer be given was that it was *so effective* that it had eradicated smallpox from the United States. In fact, within twenty years the vaccine eradicated smallpox from the world.

We should not give rubella vaccine to adult women because a study showed that 25 percent of women who received the vaccine developed a temporary arthritis.

This is a classic example of selective science. What is missing is the results of the companion study, which showed that the natural disease produced arthritis 50 percent of the time.

BE AN INFORMED CONSUMER

Your practitioner is required to give you a vaccine pamphlet for the DPT, polio, and MMR vaccines at each visit when the vaccines are given. Read them: they are very informative, describing specific symptoms and ailments that may be due to the administration of a vaccine.

If you *do* think your child has been injured by a vaccine, you can obtain information and possible compensation from:

National Vaccine Injury Compensation Program
Health Resources and Services Administration
Parklawn Building, Room 8-05
5600 Fishers Lane
Rockville, MD 20857
Telephone: (800) 338-2382

The Vaccines

MEASLES, MUMPS AND RUBELLA (MMR)

The MMR vaccine is a live virus vaccine combining three components: the vaccines against measles, mumps, and rubella (German measles). All three are the genuine disease virus weakened through repeated passage through tissue culture. They cause an immune response that is identical to that triggered by the natural disease, yet with greatly reduced side effects.

Side Effects of MMR. The MMR vaccine is administered by injection under the skin. Because the vaccine works by causing an infection, the side effects occur when the infection takes hold, not on the day of injection. At the time of injection, you can expect your child to experience a moderate burning sensation lasting only a few minutes.

The Measles Component. The effectiveness of the measles component of the vaccine is 95 percent, meaning that 95 percent of the children given the vaccine in the recommended manner develop sufficient antibodies to protect them from disease. Since 1963, when the vaccine was introduced, the incidence of measles has dropped 95 percent. A second immunization was recently added to decrease the rate of measles to a level where it would die out. As a result of this second dose, many states no longer have measles within their borders.

Side Effects of the Measles Component.

Common side effects are:

- A temperature of over 103 degrees Fahrenheit may begin seven to twelve days after vaccination and last one to two days. Approximately 5 to 15 percent of children experience this side effect.

Uncommon side effects are:

- A simple, benign febrile fit or convulsion with fever. (This is due to the fever, not the vaccine, and can occur in very young children due to any virus or bacteria that causes a significant elevation of the fever.)

Rare side effects are:

- Life-threatening allergic reactions.

Other Important Considerations. Individuals who have had life-threatening reactions to minute quantities of egg or to the antibiotic neomycin should receive this immunization only after consultation with an expert and only under well-controlled circumstances.

The vaccine should not be given within three months of a gamma globulin injection; gamma globulin may cause your child to be temporarily able to fight off the vaccination, and thus not be protected.

This vaccine *should* be given to children who are HIV infected, since it is both safe and protective in these children.

The vaccine should be postponed in children who are immunosuppressed from drugs like anticancer medications.

The Mumps Component. The mumps vaccine is 95 percent effective. It is now rare to see a case of mumps in the United States.

Side Effects of the Mumps Component.

Common side effects are: none.

Uncommon side effects are: none.

Rare side effects are:

- Life-threatening allergic reactions.

Other Important Considerations. Individuals who have had life-threatening reactions to minute quantities of egg or to the antibiotic neomycin should receive this immunization only after consultation with an expert and only under well-controlled circumstances.

The vaccine should not be given within three months of a gamma globulin injection; gamma globulin may cause your child to be temporarily able to fight off the vaccination and thus not be protected.

This vaccine *should* be given to children who are HIV infected, since it is both safe and protective in these children.

The vaccine should be postponed in children who are immunosuppressed from drugs like anticancer medications.

The Rubella Component. The rubella vaccine is 98 percent effective and has led to almost complete eradication of rubella in the United States. This is especially good news for pregnant women; a pregnant woman who is exposed to rubella may develop the dreaded complication of intrauterine infection, which can lead to infants born with congenital rubella syndrome. This syndrome can include mental retardation, blindness, deafness, and seizures.

Side Effects of the Rubella Component.

Common side effects are:

- A rash, fever, and/or swollen lymph glands may occur five to twelve days after the injection. Approximately 5 to 15 percent of children experience this side effect.
- Approximately 0.5 percent of children have joint pain seven to twenty-one days after injection.

Uncommon side effects are:

- Twenty-five percent of postpubertal females may experience joint pains or arthritis seven to twenty-one days after a first immunization. There may be a relationship with persistent arthritis following immunization in this specific group.

Rare side effects are:

- Temporary numbness and tingling in the arms and legs.

Other Important Considerations. Because of the risk of fetal damage from the natural infection, the vaccine should *not* be given to pregnant women. If the vaccine is inadvertently given to this group, however, the risk is very low.

The vaccine should not be given within three months of a gamma globulin injection; gamma globulin may cause your child to be temporarily able to fight off the vaccination and thus not be protected.

This vaccine *should* be given to children who are HIV

infected, since it is both safe and protective in these children.

The vaccine should be postponed in children who are immunosuppressed from drugs like anticancer medications.

POLIO VACCINES

Sabin Oral Polio Vaccine (TOPV). The oral polio vaccine is a live virus vaccine, derived from the natural polio virus, that has been passed repeatedly through tissue culture. This vaccine, which is actually a combination of the three closely related viruses that cause polio, works by causing an infection in the child's intestine in the same manner that the natural virus does. Polio is unique among childhood diseases in that it enters through the intestinal rather than the respiratory tract.

The Sabin vaccine is also unusual in that it can be contagious. Polio is an intestinal virus that is transmitted by hands or drinking water that have been contaminated with stool containing the virus. Anyone changing the diaper of a child with polio or recently vaccinated with the live polio virus can be exposed to that contagious virus. The virus poses no risk to most adults since they were immunized as children. Indeed, a healthy, unimmunized adult can actually be "vaccinated" in this way. Specifically at risk, however, are immunodeficient and immunosuppressed adults who have HIV infections or have had recent chemotherapy for cancer. Still, one or two of the adults who contract the disease each year have no predisposing factors when they are infected.

The vaccine is virtually 100 percent effective. In fact, vaccination with the Sabin vaccine has eliminated polio from this hemisphere.

Side Effects of TOPV.

Common side effects are: none.

Uncommon side effects are: none.

Rare side effects are:

- For reasons we don't understand, a very small percentage of healthy adults and children contract paralytic polio from the vaccine each year in the United States (one in 6 million doses from the first live immunization; far less from subsequent immunizations). There are no factors that predispose children to this complication, and it is not preventable.

Other Important Considerations. Because the vaccine is contagious, it should not be used in homes with immunodeficient or HIV-infected individuals.

The Salk Inactivated Polio Vaccine (IPV). The inactivated polio vaccine is made by growing polio virus in the laboratory and then killing or inactivating it. It is next mixed with chemicals that enhance its ability to produce immunity, and then given by intramuscular injection.

The IPV vaccine is highly effective, protecting virtually all individuals vaccinated. Because it is given by injection, it does not produce intestinal immunity. The intestines thus can become infected, and the individual can pass the disease on to others without the vaccinated individual becoming ill.

Side Effects of IPV.

Common side effects are: none.

Uncommon side effects are: none.

Rare side effects are: none.

Other Important Considerations. The IPV is the preferred form of immunization for adults who have never been immunized before but require the vaccine under special circumstances.

IPV is also the immunization of choice for HIV-infected or immunodeficient children, or for children who live in households where members are so affected.

WHICH TYPE OF POLIO VACCINE IS BETTER?

The choice for immunization for polio became more complicated recently when the National Committee on

Immunization Practice recommended that the first two immunizations for polio be given using killed vaccine (Salk—injectable) followed by two live (Sabin—oral) vaccines. Although the American Academy of Pediatrics Committee on Immunization was expected to follow with the same recommendation, it did not. The AAP said that any one of three regimens—all live vaccine (which has been standard medical practice for 40 years), all killed vaccine, or two killed vaccine doses followed by two live vaccines—is equally effective and can be used at the discretion of the parent and the pediatrician. As a result, we currently have a conflict between two organizations that usually agree.

Why do they disagree? Both vaccines are considered 100 percent effective but the live vaccine actually causes four adults and four children to contract polio each year. Given this risk, however small, why should the live vaccine be used at all?

The answer lies in the natural infection pattern with live vaccine. The oral (live) polio vaccine immunizes by causing an infection that mimics the natural infection without producing paralysis. As a result, the oral vaccine causes a complete immunity that includes the intestine and spreads to the rest of the body. The immunized child or adult cannot pick up the infection and pass it along. With the killed vaccine, which doesn't immunize the intestine, someone who is vaccinated can pick up the infection and pass it along to others without getting sick. Since polio is most certainly introduced into the United States by travelers, it is possible that young children who have had only the killed vaccine could become unwitting vehicles for the naturally occurring polio virus. (Most immunized adults have had the live vaccine.) The end result could be the return of the disease to the United States.

The change from completely oral vaccine to a combination regimen or all killed vaccine adds significant cost to the vaccine program. (The killed vaccine costs about $10 more per dose.) It is estimated that the combination vaccine regimen would reduce the number of vaccine-associated polio cases by one or two cases per year.

Your decision as to which vaccine regimen to use should be a joint decision with your pediatrician. We pediatricians have strong opinions on the subject and give them freely. We don't necessarily agree with one another. If you have any individuals in your household who are immunodeficient because of infection, chemotherapy, or a hereditary problem with the immune system, the killed vaccine is the universally recommended regimen. If your family is heathy, the regimen for your family will depend on your pediatrician's point of view, your tolerance of risk, and other factors such as the cost of immunization and the additional pain involved with the injectable vaccine.

Rest assured that whichever regimen you decide upon, it will be 100 percent effective.

HEMOPHILUS INFLUENZAE B VACCINE (HIB OR HIBD)

The hemophilus influenzae B Vaccine is *not* a flu shot. HIB is a bacteria that can be treated with antibiotics. Cousins of this bacteria cause sinus and ear infections. This particular bacteria, unfortunately, was the most common cause of meningitis in children, as well as epiglottitis (a life-threatening infection of the valve that closes the windpipe when you swallow) and serious skin infections in young children.

The vaccine is made from a portion of the sugar coating (polysaccharide coat) of the bacteria that is attached to a protein. It causes a child's immune system to make antibodies at an earlier age than normal.

This vaccine has been very effective. Since there are four brands of vaccine, each somewhat different, it is difficult to quote effectiveness rates—yet all four vaccines appear highly effective in producing antibodies. Most importantly,

HIB meningitis and epiglottitis are now extremely rare in vaccinated children.

Side Effects of HIB.

Common side effects are:

- Approximately 25 percent of children will have pain, redness, and/or swelling at the injection site. This is mild and lasts less than 24 hours.

Uncommon side effects are:

- Fever and irritability.

Rare side effects are: none.

Other Important Considerations. There are four brands of the vaccine, each somewhat different. Until we have further data, it is recommended that the same vaccine be used for each dose.

The number of doses decreases with the age of the child. A single dose is all that is necessary after age one.

Children over the age of five are naturally immune to HIB and do not require vaccination.

HEPATITIS B VACCINE

The hepatitis B vaccine protects against serum hepatitis, which is the most serious form of hepatitis. The vaccine is made by using a genetic engineering technique to reproduce the part of the virus coat that produces antibodies. No live virus is involved in this process, and no human products are involved. There is no possibility of infection from the vaccine.

Pediatricians have begun a program to eliminate serum hepatitis within a generation. An immunization program for infants was begun in 1992, and the vaccine is now recommended for all infants in the first year and all adolescents.

Children are given a series of three immunizations on a variable schedule. It is not known whether booster immunizations will be necessary in the future.

The vaccine produces protective antibodies in 90 to 95 percent of children immunized.

Side Effects of the Hepatitis B Vaccine.

Common side effects are:

- A low-grade fever affects 1 to 6 percent of vaccinated children.

Uncommon side effects are: none.

Rare side effects are: none.

Other Important Considerations. No serious side effects are associated with this vaccine, and no test is required before the immunization is given. Even people infected with hepatitis, presently or in the past, can be immunized without concern.

DIPHTHERIA, PERTUSSIS, AND TETANUS VACCINE (DPT)

The diphtheria, pertussis, and tetanus (DPT) vaccine was developed to vaccinate against three diseases caused by bacteria that cause damage by the toxins they produce. In all three cases, treating and killing the bacteria that cause the disease has little effect on the disease, because the toxins are still produced.

The vaccine is available as:

- Diphtheria + tetanus
- Diphtheria + pertussis + tetanus
- Diphtheria + pertussis + tetanus + hemophilus influenzae
- Diptheria + acellular pertussis + tetanus

All combinations work equally well. Here we discuss the diphtheria and tetanus vaccine together, followed by a separate exploration of the more controversial pertussis vaccine. (The hemophilus influenzae vaccine has already been discussed above.)

Diphtheria and Tetanus Vaccine. The diphtheria and tetanus vaccines are toxoids. That is, the vaccine is against the toxins produced by diphtheria and tetanus bacteria. Diphtheria is only found in humans, and is passed from one infected person to another. Tetanus is a common organism found in the soil and is present in "dirty" wounds. The vaccine is a killed vaccine.

The diphtheria vaccine has virtually eliminated diphtheria in the United States. Those cases of diphtheria that currently occur (about five cases yearly) do so in older people who have not been immunized.

The tetanus vaccine offers virtually complete protection. Tetanus does not occur in children who have been immunized against this disease.

The vaccines should be given every ten years throughout adulthood to ensure lifetime protection.

Side Effects.

Common side effects are:

- Local pain, swelling, and low-grade temperature.

Uncommon side effects are: none.

Rare side effects are: none.

Other Important Considerations. Diphtheria vaccines for adults and children are distinctly different. Adults given the children's vaccine tend to have intense inflammation of the muscles, and are therefore given doses that are one third to one sixth as strong as children's vaccines.

Pertussis Vaccine (Whooping Cough). The pertussis vaccine is produced in two forms. The traditional vaccine is the crudest vaccine in use. It consists of the whole pertussis bacteria, killed and mixed with a substance that improves its ability to produce antibodies.

The second form of the vaccine, called acellular pertussis vaccine, was developed in Japan and has only a portion of the outer coat of the bacteria. The acellular vaccine is much less likely to cause side effects, both minor and major. The acellular pertussis vaccine was recently approved for use in children of all ages and should be the preferred vaccine.

The acellular pertussis vaccine is 80 to 85 percent effective. This is significantly better than the original vaccine. Immunity decreases after three years.

Children who have been vaccinated against pertussis can still become infected, but generally have mild or inapparent disease. When 70 percent of the children in a population have been immunized, epidemic pertussis, which is associated with the highest fatality rates, does not occur.

Approximately 30 percent of children who are not immunized are diagnosed with pertussis. Pertussis occurs frequently during the winter as a mild illness in school-age children and adults and is often not diagnosed.

Side Effects of the Pertussis Vaccine.

The common side effects described below have been almost completely eliminated by the acellular pertussis vaccine and should not be routinely expected with the new acellular vaccine. Rare side effects will most likely also be reduced or eliminated, but it is too soon to be certain if this will occur.

Common side effects of traditional (whole) vaccine are:

- Redness, edema, induration, and tenderness at the injection site.
- Drowsiness, fretfulness, loss of appetite, vomiting, crying and mild to moderate fever (lower than 103.5 degrees Fahrenheit).

Uncommon side effects are:

- Hives may occur, but are not a particularly serious side effect.

Rare side effects are:

- Allergic reactions to the vaccine can occur. A severe, life-threatening allergic reaction can occur in 2 out of 100,000 injections.

More About Serious Side Effects. Side effects of the pertussis vaccine are common, and there are also serious adverse reactions that deserve special mention. While side effects can occur with *any* form of the vaccine, they are much more common with the traditional whole cell pertussis vaccine than with the newer acellular vaccine.

- Unusual crying: Persistent, severe, inconsolable screaming or crying for three or more hours within forty-eight hours of immunization. There is no specific known cause for this reaction. The crying is alarming to parents, but does not appear to cause any permanent injury to children.
- Collapse: Occasionally (1 in 1750 doses), an infant will lose muscle tone and turn pale. An infant in this state is often described as a "rag doll." Fortunately, there appear to be no long-term consequences from this reaction.
- Seizures: Occasionally (1 in 1750 doses), the pertussis vaccine will cause a fever (often over 105 degrees Fahrenheit), which triggers a convulsion. These convulsions are considered to be "benign febrile convulsions" that are brief, do not lead to permanent injury, and do not predispose the infant to further seizures. On very rare occasions it is possible that the fever may trigger a more severe seizure, with the risk of possible long-term disability. Yet, data on this is sparse, and it is not clear just how often, if ever, this occurs.

Caution: If any one of these reactions occur, the pertussis vaccination should either not be given again or should be given only with the advice and under the supervision of experts.

Other Important Considerations. There has been no evidence linking sudden infant death syndrome (SIDS) or a disease called infantile spasms with the pertussis vaccine.

The best designed studies have shown no relationship between pertussis vaccine and the development of severe neurologic illness in children.

Parents of infants with neurologic disorders or a previous history of convulsion should consult with their pediatrician before vaccinating against pertussis.

Immunization Update

Our current vaccines are not perfect. We need vaccines with fewer side effects and better and more lasting immunity. A faster and more efficient system is also required to approve new vaccines and detect problems with vaccines that are already licensed.

Better immunizations worldwide would result in the elimination of disease, eventually rendering many immunizations themselves obsolete. Smallpox has been eradicated through immunization, and polio no longer exists in our hemisphere because of the oral polio vaccine. The elimination of disease is only possible through immunization, and that is the ultimate goal of our immunization program.

5

THE MOST COMMON PRESCRIPTION DRUGS FOR CHILDREN

In this chapter you will find an accessible and easy-to-use A-to-Z guide to the medications most frequently prescribed for children. Prescription drugs are alphabetized by their generic name, which is the same as their primary active ingredient. But before examining each individual medication, let's take a closer look at the types of drugs most often prescribed by pediatricians.

ANTI-ASTHMA MEDICATIONS

Asthma is the most common chronic disease of childhood, and the narrow airways in the lungs of very small children are most susceptible to obstruction. Left untreated, asthma can be a severe and even life-threatening condition.

There are two primary types of anti-asthma medications. The routine use of anti-inflammatory drugs (such as beclomethasone and cromolyn sodium) can help prevent the inflammation that leads to the symptoms of asthma, while bronchodilators (albuterol, theophylline, etcetera) relax the small, smooth muscles that tighten around a child's airways and constrict breathing.

An important part of asthma management is identifying and removing the triggers of asthma. Bronchodilators should not allow you to continue to expose your child to allergens, irritants, and other airborne substances that can damage his or her lungs.

ANTIBIOTICS

Antibiotics are prescribed to treat a wide range of bacterial diseases in children, including middle ear, respiratory, urinary tract, and skin infections. They are only effective against bacterial—not víral, parasitic, or fungal—infections. Antibiotics destroy bacteria but do not harm human cells.

If your child does not show signs of improvement following treatment with one antibiotic, consult your pediatrician. Your child may be suffering from an infection that is resistant to that antibiotic. For example, amoxicillin is most often effective for ear infections, erythromycin is most appropriate for mild to moderate infections, and antibiotics such as clindamycin and metronidazole are prescribed in serious infections caused by the most drug-resistant bacteria.

For treatment with antibiotics to be effective—and to prevent infection from recurring—it's important to follow the entire course of medication prescribed by your pediatrician, even after your child's symptoms have diminished or disappeared.

ANTICONVULSANTS

Anticonvulsant drugs are commonly prescribed to treat and prevent seizure disorders in children. Yet, a greater scientific understanding of their effects has led to changes in their use over the last few years.

In the recent past, phenobarbital was very commonly prescribed for febrile (nonepileptic) seizures in children. Febrile seizures can occur in children between three months and five years of age, and are usually due to a rapid rise or fall in body temperature, rather than simply a high fever. Contrary to popular opinion, febrile seizures, while alarming to parents, do not cause brain damage in children. As a result, most children with febrile seizures are no longer medicated.

Because phenobarbital interferes with learning and can cause behavior problems, its use is now limited to infants. Other drugs, such as valproic acid and carbamazepine, are more commonly used for children with recurrent seizures. Chronic use of seizure medication (for more than 2 years) is reserved for special situations. If your child has been prescribed seizure medications such as phenobarbital for more than 2 years without EEG (brain wave) testing, consult a pediatric neurologist to determine if these drugs are needed.

ANTIHISTAMINES

Antihistamines work by blocking the action of histamine released from specialized allergy cells called mast cells. Histamine is the substance that most commonly causes itching and inflammation, and reactions to histamine can lead to difficulty in breathing due to narrowing and inflammation of the airways and increased mucous secretion.

Antihistamines can also control sensitive or allergic reactions when your child's skin comes into contact with potential irritants, such as harsh chemicals in detergents or nickel in jewelry. They may be prescribed when your child experiences penicillin sensitivity or an allergic reaction to certain foods.

Oral antihistamines are especially helpful when topical products alone are insufficient to control itching and inflammation. They help control itching due to an allergic reaction, hives, chicken pox, and atopic dermatitis (eczema).

ATTENTION DEFICIT HYPERACTIVITY DISORDER (ADHD) MEDICATIONS

Central nervous system stimulants are prescribed to treat the behavioral syndrome known as attention deficit hyperactivity disorder (ADHD) in children. They act to calm the hyperactive child, contributing to the management of overactivity and lengthening the attention spans of hyperactive children. Drugs that are used to manage attention deficit disorders should be integrated within a complete program of psychological, social, and educational treatment.

CORTICOSTEROIDS

Under the letter "C" we have included a combination profile of a very important group of prescription drugs: topical corticosteroids. Some of the weaker corticosteroids included in this group profile are also available in over-the-counter forms. We have grouped these widely used medications together because they have similar effects on your child's body and thus are used to treat similar infections. Through examining the charts on pages 105–107 you can better understand and compare the various strengths, functions, and side effects of these medications, and determine with your pediatrician which, if any, are right for your child.

In each of the profiles that follow you will find:

- General information about the medication
- What type of dosage is appropriate for your child
- How to best administer the medication, such as with or without food or at a particular time of day
- How often to administer the medication
- What common side effects to keep an eye out for
- More serious adverse reactions that may warrant discontinuing the medication and consulting your pediatrician
- Important precautions such as drug interactions

Below we list generic names with which you may be familiar. If you want to look up a product by brand name, turn to the index.

Prescription Drugs

Acyclovir
Albuterol
Alclometasone Dipropionate
Amcinonide
Amoxicillin
Amoxicillin with Clavulanic Acid
Antipyrine and Benzocaine Glycerin
Azithromycin
Beclomethasone
Betamethasone
Betamethasone Dipropionate
Betamethasone Valerate
Brompheniramine Maleate, Phenylpropanolamine Hydrochloride, and Codeine
Carbamazepine
Cefaclor
Cefadroxil
Cefixime
Cefprozil
Cephalexin
Cephradine
Chloral Hydrate
Cimetidine
Clarithromycin
Clindamycin
Clobetasol Propionate
Codeine
Corticosteroids, Topical
Cromolyn
Cyproheptadine
Desmopressin Acetate
Desonide
Desoximetasone
Dexamethasone
Dexamethasone Phosphate
Dextroamphetamine
Dicloxacillin
Diflorasone Diacetate
Diphenoxylate Hydrochloride with Atropine Sulfate
Doxycycline
Erythromycin (Oral)
Erythromycin (Eye Medication)
Erythromycin Ethylsuccinate and Sulfisoxazole Acetyl
Flunisolide
Fluocinolone Acetonide
Fluocinonide
Fluoride with Vitamins and Minerals
Flurandrenolide

Gamma Benzene Hexachloride
Griseofulvin
Guaifenesin, Pseudoephedrine, and Codeine
Halcinonide
Hydrocortisone Valerate
Hydroxyzine
Hyoscyamine Sulfate, Atropine Sulfate, Scopolamine Hydrobromide, and Phenobarbital
Imipramine
Isoniazid
Ketoconazole
Lidocaine
Loracarbef
Mebendazole
Methylphenidate
Methylprednisolone
Methylprednisone Acetate
Metronidazole
Minocycline
Mupirocin
Nitrofurantoin
Nystatin
Pemoline
Penicillin V Potassium
Phenobarbital
Phenytoin
Polymyxin B, Neomycin Sulfate, and Gramicidin (Eye Medication)
Polymyxin B, Neomycin Sulfate, and Hydrocortisone (Eardrops)
Prednisone
Prochlorperazine
Promethazine
Ranitidine
Sulfacetamide (Eye Medication)
Sulfisoxazole (Oral)
Sulfisoxazole (Eye Medication)
Tetracycline
Theophylline
Tobramycin (Eye Medication)
Triamcinolone and Nystatin
Triamcinolone Acetonide
Trimethoprim and Sulfamethoxazole
Valproic Acid

ACYCLOVIR

BRAND NAME
Zovirax

GENERAL INFORMATION
Acyclovir is generally prescribed to treat infections caused by herpes viruses, which include chicken pox in children. Acyclovir works by interfering with the reproduction of the virus. While there is no cure for chicken pox or other herpes viruses, treatment with acyclovir can reduce pain and help sores heal faster if started within 24 hours of the breakout.

DOSAGE AND ADMINISTRATION
Treatment with acyclovir should be initiated as soon as your child clearly shows symptoms of chicken pox, within the first 24 hours of disease. Acyclovir is available for children in suspension, capsule, and tablet form. Administer four times a day, and do not exceed 3200 mg in a 24-hour period. Your physician may adjust the dosage for children who fall in-between the following weights. The dosages given below are specifically for the treatment of chicken pox.

	200 mg suspension	200 mg capsules	800 mg tablets
12 lb	½ tsp	—	—
22 lb	1 tsp	—	—
33 lb	1½ tsp	—	—
44 lb	2 tsp	2	—
66 lb	3 tsp	3	—
88 lb	—	4	1

SIDE EFFECTS
Treatment with acyclovir does not usually cause side effects.

Infrequently, adverse reactions include fluid retention, nausea, and vomiting. If your child experiences any of these effects, discontinue use at once and consult your pediatrician.

IMPORTANT PRECAUTIONS

For treatment with acyclovir to be effective, it is important to start treatment immediately and follow the entire course of medication prescribed by your pediatrician. Acyclovir should not be given to children who have experienced a sensitivity or allergic reaction to it in the past.

ALBUTEROL

BRAND NAMES

Proventil, Ventolin

GENERAL INFORMATION

Albuterol is prescribed to relieve the obstruction of upper airways that occurs in asthma. Asthma is the most common chronic disease of childhood, and the narrow airways in the lungs of very small children are most susceptible to obstruction. Left untreated, asthma can be a severe and even life-threatening condition.

Albuterol is a member of a class of asthma-relieving medications known as bronchodilators, which act by relaxing the small, smooth muscles that tighten around a child's airways and constrict breathing. Albuterol provides fast and effective relief of asthma symptoms.

DOSAGE AND ADMINISTRATION

Albuterol is most commonly inhaled into the lungs through either metered-dose inhalers or nebulizers. Breathing in medication is an effective way of getting it directly to the airways.

Metered-dose inhalers, or MDIs, can be used by children once they are ten years old. An MDI is a small hand-held device from which the appropriate dose of medication is released into the mouth as the child breathes in. Spacer devices (Aerochamber, Inspirease) are now coming into general use and allow MDIs to be used to treat even very young children. This is both effective and convenient for parents.

Nebulizers are an easier way to deliver medication to small children. In this method, medication is placed in a small canister attached to a face mask and then nebulized into a fine mist, which can be easily inhaled.

Albuterol in syrup form can be useful in young children with mild symptoms. Tablets, while available, are now rarely used.

	Syrup* (every 6–8 hours)	Solution for inhalation (as directed)	Inhaler (every 4–6 hours or as directed)	Tablets
12 lb	½ tsp	0.2 cc	—	—
22 lb	1 tsp	0.4 cc	—	—
33 lb	1½ tsp	0.5 cc***	1–2 puffs	—
44 lb	2 tsp	0.5 cc***	as above	use inhaled medication
66 lb	**	0.5 cc***	as above	use inhaled medication
88 lb	**	0.5 cc***	as above	use inhaled medication

*The dosage may be cut in half and still remain effective the first few times the medication is given.

**Inhaled medications are used at this weight.

***May be given using dropper with normal saline or cromolyn, or as a unit dose vial.

SIDE EFFECTS

The most common side effects of treatment with albuterol are a tremor and rapid heartbeat. Albuterol sometimes interferes with falling asleep. If this happens, give the medication at bedtime when your child is already sleepy.

Less common but more serious adverse reactions include dizziness, anxiety and nervousness, and overstimulation. If your child experiences any of these effects, discontinue use at once and consult your pediatrician. A lower dose may be all that is needed to prevent side effects.

IMPORTANT PRECAUTIONS

Because bronchodilators such as albuterol are used to control the outward symptoms of asthma, you may be lulled into a false sense of security about your child's well-being. By relieving uncomfortable symptoms, albuterol may allow you to continue to expose your child to allergens, irritants, and other airborne substances that can damage his or her lungs.

Albuterol should not be used every day as the sole asthma medication. Preventive medications (such as cromolyn or inhaled steroids) should be given with albuterol if daily medication is required.

If a standard 200-dose inhaler does not last for 30 days, consult your pediatrician to review your child's medications.

ALCLOMETASONE DIPROPIONATE

See Corticosteroids, Topical

AMCINONIDE

See Corticosteroids, Topical

AMOXICILLIN

BRAND NAMES

Amoxil, Larotid, Polymox, Trimox, Wymox

GENERAL INFORMATION

Amoxicillin is a penicillin antibiotic commonly prescribed to treat a wide range of bacterial infections, including middle ear infections, infections of the upper and lower respiratory tract, urinary tract infections, and skin infections. Amoxicillin is the most frequently prescribed drug for young children, since it is inexpensive, tastes good (like pink bubble gum), and is effective for most young children's infections. Even though 20 to 30 percent of bacteria may be resistant to amoxicillin, it remains the drug of choice for ear infections because of its many positive qualities.

Inside your child's body, amoxicillin is converted into ampicillin, the effective drug. Yet amoxicillin is better absorbed into the body than ampicillin, and causes fewer side effects (such as nonallergic rashes and diarrhea). Amoxicillin kills infectious bacteria by invading and damaging bacterial cell walls, causing the susceptible bacteria to fall apart. Yet it has no effect on human cell walls, which are made differently.

Amoxicillin, like other antibiotics, is only effective against susceptible bacterial—not viral, parasitic, or fungal—infections. Your child will usually show signs of improvement following one to two days of treatment, and should be well on the road to recovery in three to four days. If toxic symptoms or discomfort continue after this time, consult your pediatrician. Your child may be suffering from an infection that is resistant to amoxicillin, in which case the doctor may want to see your child and/or prescribe an alternate treatment.

DOSAGE AND ADMINISTRATION

Amoxicillin is available for children in pediatric drops, oral suspension, and chewable tablets. The liquid forms are usually preferable for younger children. Refrigeration of the suspension is not required, but amoxicillin tastes better when refrigerated, which makes it easier for your child to swallow. Containers of amoxicillin should be kept tightly closed and protected from light.

Amoxicillin should be administered three times a day. The dosages below are calculated at 18–23 mg per pound. Doses as low as 10 mg per pound are recommended but are unlikely to be effective for most uses. Your physician may adjust the dosage for children who fall in-between the following weights.

	Pediatric drops	125 mg suspension	250 mg suspension	125 mg chewable	250 mg chewable	Capsules–250–500 mg
12 lb	1.8 cc	¾ tsp	—	—	—	—
22 lb	—	1⅓ tsp	½–⅔ tsp	1	—	—
33 lb	—	2 tsp	1 tsp	2	1	—
44 lb	—	2–2½ tsp	1–1⅓ tsp	2	1	—
66 lb	—	—	1⅔–2 tsp	—	2	250–500 mg
88 lb	—	—	2 tsp	—	2	500 mg

SIDE EFFECTS

The most common side effects of treatment with amoxicillin are allergic skin rashes. Allergic reactions to amoxicillin are most likely to occur after the initial week of treatment, and within the first twenty-four hours in patients who have had allergic reactions previously. If a skin rash becomes severe, discontinue use and consult your pediatrician.

Less common but more serious adverse reactions include hives, swelling of the body, joint pain, and swollen lymph nodes. If your child experiences any of these effects, discontinue use at once and consult your pediatrician.

In rare cases of respiratory difficulty or shock, take your child to the emergency room immediately.

IMPORTANT PRECAUTIONS

For treatment with amoxicillin to be effective—and to prevent infection from recurring—it's important to follow the entire course of medication prescribed by your pediatrician, even after your child's symptoms have diminished or disappeared.

Amoxicillin should be used with caution in children who have a history of severe allergic reactions to many substances. A minor dotlike rash, especially one that occurs two to four days after treatment has begun, is more likely to be viral than allergic. Hives that appear after each dose, on the other hand, are probably allergic reactions. If the reaction is mild, your pediatrician may try amoxicillin again at a later date. If your child has had a severe reaction to amoxicillin or penicillin, cephalosporins should be given with close medical supervision.

AMOXICILLIN WITH CLAVULANIC ACID

BRAND NAME

Augmentin

GENERAL INFORMATION

Augmentin is prescribed to treat lower respiratory infections, middle ear infections, and sinus, skin, and urinary tract infections that are caused by specific bacteria. Augmentin combines clavulanic acid and amoxicillin to "augment" the effectiveness of the antibiotic amoxicillin. Clavulanic acid attaches itself to an enzyme known as beta lactamase, which can chop amoxicillin into ineffective pieces. Once attached, it won't detach. This renders the beta lactamase ineffective and allows amoxicillin to kill many bacteria that would normally be resistant to it.

Like other antibiotics, Augmentin is effective against many susceptible *bacterial*—not viral, parasitic or fungal—infections. Your child will usually respond to treatment within several days. If he or she continues to experience fever or pain after this time, consult your pediatrician. Your child may be suffering from an infection that is resistant to Augmentin, in which case the doctor may want to see your child and/or prescribe an alternate treatment.

DOSAGE AND ADMINISTRATION

Because the clavulanic acid irritates the intestine in approximately 20 percent of children, Augmentin must be taken with water or food. Augmentin is available for children in pediatric drops, suspension, and chewable tablets. The liquid forms are preferable for younger children.

Doses of Augmentin are usually administered three times a day. (A new formulation has become available allowing for twice daily dosages. Ask your physician if this more convenient regimen is appropriate for your child.) Published dosage range is calculated at 9–18 mg per pound. These dosages are calculated at the higher range, which is more likely to be effective. Your physician may adjust the dosage for children who fall in-between the following weights.

3 TIMES DAILY DOSAGE REGIMEN

	125 mg suspension	250 mg suspension	125 mg chewable tablets	250 mg chewable tablets	250 mg tablets	500 mg tablets
12 lb	⅔ tsp	—	—	—	—	—
22 lb	1 tsp	½ tsp	1	—	—	—
33 lb	1½–1⅔ tsp	¾ tsp	1	—	—	—
44 lb	2 tsp	1 tsp	2	1	—	—
66 lb	—	1⅔	—	1½	1	—
88 lb	—	2	—	2	1*	1

*Because the dose of clavulanic acid is the same in both strengths of tablets, two 250 mg tablets cannot be used in the place of one 500 mg tablet without causing significant gastrointestinal discomfort.

SIDE EFFECTS

Common side effects of treatment with Augmentin include diarrhea, flatulence, headache, nausea, upset stomach, and vaginitis. If one or more of these complaints become severe, discontinue use and consult your pediatrician.

A less common but more serious adverse reaction is hives. If your child experiences this effect, discontinue use at once and consult your pediatrician.

IMPORTANT PRECAUTIONS

For treatment with Augmentin to be effective—and to prevent infection from recurring—it's important to follow the entire course of medication prescribed by your pediatrician (usually ten to fourteen days), even after your child's symptoms have diminished or disappeared.

Augmentin should not be given to children who have a history of allergic reactions to amoxicillin, penicillin, or cephalosporin antibiotics (such as Ceclor).

Augmentin should be used with caution in children who have a history of multiple allergies, asthma, hay fever, or hives.

ANTIPYRINE AND BENZOCAINE GLYCERIN

BRAND NAMES

Auralgan Ear Drops, Auroto Otic

GENERAL INFORMATION

This combination medication, commonly known as Auralgan Ear Drops, is prescribed to relieve the pain and discomfort of middle ear infections. The analgesic action of prescription Auralgan is more effective than over-the-counter acetaminophen in relieving ear pain caused by the pressure, inflammation, and congestion that often accompany middle ear infections. This drug is often prescribed in combination with an antibiotic to treat painful middle ear infections, since Auralgan relieves pain while antibiotics kill the underlying bacteria that are causing the infection.

DOSAGE AND ADMINISTRATION

Auralgan should be administered every two hours as needed for pain. Apply the medication drop by drop until the ear canal is filled, using the dropper provided with the medicine and trying not to touch the ear with the dropper. After use, gently place a sterile cotton ball or piece of gauze in the outer ear. Do not rinse the dropper after application, and replace Auralgan six months after the original use of the medication.

SIDE EFFECTS

While local irritation and allergic reactions are not usual reactions to treatment with Auralgan, discontinue use and consult your pediatrician if your child experiences these effects. Serious side effects to Auralgan are unknown.

IMPORTANT PRECAUTIONS

Auralgan should not be given to children who have a history of allergic reactions to any of the ingredients in Auralgan or similar medications.

AZITHROMYCIN

BRAND NAME

Zithromax

GENERAL INFORMATION

Azithromycin is a new antibiotic related to erythromycin. Prescribed to treat respiratory tract infections, mild skin problems, and strep throat, it has recently been approved for use in children over the age of six months.

Like other antibiotics, azithromycin is effective against many susceptible *bacterial*—not viral, parasitic or fungal—infections. Your child will usually respond to treatment within a day or two. If he or she continues to experience fever or pain after this time, consult your pediatrician. Your child may be suffering from an infection that is resistant to azithromycin, in which case the doctor may want to see your child and/or prescribe an alternate treatment.

DOSAGE AND ADMINISTRATION

Azithromycin is an unusual drug in that it is given for only five days and yet it has the effect of ten days of other medications. Ordinarily, the first dose is a double dose, to be given on an empty stomach. A special feature of this medication is that a different dosage is used for strep throat.

REGULAR DOSAGE

	100 mg/tsp suspension	200 mg/tsp suspension	250 mg capsules
12 lb	½ tsp/¼ tsp	—	—
22 lb	1 tsp/½ tsp	—	—
33 lb	—	¾ tsp/½ tsp	—
44 lb	—	1 tsp/½ tsp	—
66 lb	—	1½ tsp/¾ tsp	—
88 lb	—	2½ tsp/1¼ tsp	2/1

Note: The initial dose is listed first, followed by the subsequent daily doses.

DOSAGE FOR STREPTOCOCCAL SORE THROAT

	100 mg/tsp suspension	200 mg/tsp suspension	250 mg capsules
12 lb	⅔ tsp*	⅓ tsp*	—
22 lb	1¼	⅔ tsp	—
33 lb	—	1 tsp	—
44 lb	—	1½ tsp	—
66 lb	—	2 tsp	—
88 lb	—	2½ tsp/1¼	2/1

*Treatment of streptococcal sore throat below two years of age is controversial.

Note: When treating a streptococcal sore throat, the dosage is the same for each of the five days of treatment except for 88 lb, where the dosage is halved on days 2–5.

SIDE EFFECTS

The most common side effects of treatment with azithromycin are cramps, diarrhea, and nausea. If one or more of these complaints become severe, discontinue use and consult your pediatrician.

Less common adverse reactions include dizziness, drowsiness, headache, heart palpitations, indigestion, jaundice, and allergic reactions. If your child experiences any of these effects, discontinue use at once and consult your pediatrician.

IMPORTANT PRECAUTIONS

For treatment with azithromycin to be effective—and to prevent infection from recurring—it's important to follow the entire course of medication prescribed by your pediatrician, even after your child's symptoms have diminished or disappeared.

Azithromycin should not be given to children who have a history of allergic reactions to erythromycin.

Since azithromycin causes heightened light sensitivity, limit your child's exposure to sunlight or apply a broad-based sunscreen before going outside.

BECLOMETHASONE

BRAND NAMES
Beclovent, Vanceril

GENERAL INFORMATION
Beclomethasone is a corticosteroid medication prescribed to prevent the symptoms of asthma. Because it is a preventive anti-inflammatory drug, beclomethasone reduces inflammation in the lungs, which means both fewer asthmatic episodes and a reduced possibility of permanent lung damage due to asthma.

DOSAGE AND ADMINISTRATION
Beclomethasone is inhaled into the lungs through either metered-dose inhalers or nebulizers. Breathing in medication is an effective way of getting it directly to the airways.

Metered-dose inhalers, or MDIs, can be used by children using spacer devices (Aerochamber, Inspirease), at a very young age. An MDI is a small hand-held device from which the appropriate dose of medication is released into the mouth as the child breathes in.

Nebulizers are another way to deliver medication to small children. In this method, medication is placed in a small canister attached to a face mask and then nebulized into a fine mist, which can be easily inhaled.

Beclomethasone is normally administered twice a day. The dosage does not vary with weight or age.

SIDE EFFECTS
The most common side effects of treatment with beclomethasone are dry mouth, hoarseness, and sore throat. Rinsing the mouth after using is an easy way to prevent most side effects.

Less common adverse reactions include yeast infections of the mouth or larynx, which are characterized by a persistent sensitive throat. If your child experiences one of these problems, consult your pediatrician.

IMPORTANT PRECAUTIONS

Beclomethasone is a preventive medication and is not appropriate for the treatment of asthma attacks; your child will probably require a separate bronchodilator medication (such as albuterol) for this purpose.

Because beclomethasone is a preventive, anti-inflammatory medication, results may not be evident for one to two weeks after treatment has begun. Nevertheless, in order for beclomethasone to be effective, doses should be continued on a regular basis as prescribed by your pediatrician. Only your pediatrician should make adjustments in dosage.

When administering both bronchodilator and beclomethasone medications to control your child's asthma, the bronchodilator should be given first in order to optimize the effectiveness of the beclomethasone.

BETAMETHASONE

BRAND NAME

Diprolene

GENERAL INFORMATION

Betamethasone is a topical anti-inflammatory corticosteroid prescribed to relieve skin rashes in children. These itchy, irritating, and often oozing rashes include eczema, contact dermatitis (a rash due to contact with irritants ranging from poison ivy to detergents used to wash clothing to nickel in jewelry), and psoriasis.

While the exact causes of most rashes remain unknown, certain children appear especially prone to developing them, probably due to genetic predisposition. Identifying and avoiding the substance or substances that trigger rashes is important, as is keeping your child's fingernails well-clipped when rashes develop.

Depending on the severity of the rash, your pediatrician will recommend an over-the-counter product such as hydrocortisone ½ to 1% (CaldeCORT or Cortaid), prescribe a mild topical corticosteroid preparation such as fluocinonide, or a stronger one such as betamethasone. (For a comprehensive discussion of topical corticosteroids, turn to page 102.)

DOSAGE AND ADMINISTRATION

Betamethasone is available in cream, lotion, and ointment form. Apply once or twice daily, as directed by your pediatrician. A thin film is sufficient, and treated skin should ideally be left exposed to the air, or at most, loosely covered. Never cover with tight bandages unless specifically directed by your doctor.

SIDE EFFECTS

The most common side effect of treatment with betamethasone is thinning of the skin, especially when it is used on sensitive areas such as the face, neck, or genitals. Use the smallest effective amount to protect the skin.

Less common but more serious adverse reactions include persistent redness or raised bumps on the skin, which may indicate skin disorders such as acne, rosacea, miliaria, or folliculitis. A rare but potentially very serious complication of treatment with topical corticosteroids over large areas of the body is Cushing's syndrome; this is a serious disease characterized by depression, mood swings, high blood pressure, insomnia, water retention, weight gain, round face, and muscle weakness. If your child experiences any of these effects, discontinue use at once and consult your pediatrician.

IMPORTANT PRECAUTIONS

While betamethasone is very effective in relieving skin rashes, even small amounts can be absorbed through the skin and disrupt adrenal function. This is an especially serious concern for children, since the production of growth hormones may be disrupted.

The single most important thing to remember when using betamethasone in children is to use it for a short period of time (approximately one week) unless specifically instructed by a pediatrician or dermatologist. Apply betamethasone only as directed by your pediatrician and use it sparingly.

Betamethasone is for external use only. Do not apply it in the sensitive area around your child's eyes.

BETAMETHASONE DIPROPIONATE

See Corticosteroids, Topical

BETAMETHASONE VALERATE

See Corticosteroids, Topical

BROMPHENIRAMINE MALEATE, PHENYLPROPANOLAMINE HYDROCHLORIDE, AND CODEINE

BRAND NAME

Dimetane Cough Syrup AC

GENERAL INFORMATION

Dimetane Cough Syrup AC is prescribed to relieve cough and cold symptoms in children. It is very effective in drying congestion and controlling coughs. However, since codeine is serious medicine for children, your pediatrician will usually recommend that you try over-the-counter products before turning to Dimetane AC. (For more information about cough and cold preparations, turn to page 239.)

DOSAGE AND ADMINISTRATION

Dimetane Cough Syrup AC is not recommended for children under age one. It should be administered three to four times a day as needed for a one-week period. Your physician may adjust the dosage for children who fall in-between the following weights.

12 lb	Not recommended
22 lb	¼–½ tsp every 4–6 hours
33 lb	½–¾ tsp every 4–6 hours
44 lb	½–1 tsp every 4–6 hours
66 lb	1–1½ tsp every 4–6 hours
88 lb	1–2 tsp every 4–6 hours

SIDE EFFECTS

The most common side effects of treatment with Dimetane Cough Syrup AC are sleepiness, dry mouth and throat, dizziness, and constipation. If one or more of these complaints become severe, discontinue use and consult your pediatrician.

Less common serious side effects or adverse reactions include nausea and vomiting. If your child experiences any of these effects, discontinue use at once and consult your pediatrician.

IMPORTANT PRECAUTIONS

Dimetane Cough Syrup AC is a powerful medication and should be administered with care. Large doses of products that contain codeine can lead to respiratory depression, while long-term use of codeine causes physical dependence. This cough syrup should be used with care in children who have asthma, diabetes, heart problems, or thyroid disease.

CARBAMAZEPINE

BRAND NAMES

Atretol, Epitol, Tegretol

GENERAL INFORMATION

Carbamazepine is an anticonvulsant drug prescribed for the treatment of seizure disorders in children. In fact, carbamazepine is often the medication of choice for children in many situations. It also has an antidepressant effect and may be helpful in the management of behavioral disorders in children. Yet, since it has potentially serious side effects, it should be used with discretion.

DOSAGE AND ADMINISTRATION

Carbamazepine is administered to children three to four times a day, after a gradual introduction. It is available in suspension and tablet form. Your physican may adjust the dosage for children who fall in-between the weights in the chart on page 80.

SIDE EFFECTS

Common side effects include drowsiness, dizziness, nausea, and vomiting during initial treatment with carbamazepine (Tegretol). Their impact may be diminished by cutting dosage. *Other side effects* include confusion, headache, fatigue,

	100 mg/tsp suspension	100 mg chewable tabs	200 mg tablets
12 lb	1/8–1/2 tsp twice daily	—	—
22 lb	1/4–1 tsp twice daily	—	—
33 lb	1/3–1 1/2 tsp twice daily	1/2–1 1/2 tablets twice daily	—
44 lb	1/2–2 tsp twice daily	1/2–2 tablets twice daily	—
66 lb	3/4–3 tsp twice daily	1–3 tablets twice daily	1/2–1 1/2 tablets twice daily
88 lb	1–4 tsp twice daily	1–4 tablets twice daily	1/2–2 tablets twice daily

and diplopia (double vision). If one or more of these complaints become severe, discontinue use and consult your pediatrician.

There is a potential risk of very serious and even life-threatening side effects in children who are given carbamazepine. Severe dermatological reactions, ranging from hives to Stevens Johnson syndrome, a severe skin disorder, occasionally occur. In addition, rare but very serious problems such as blood disorders, cardiovascular irregularities, and metabolic reactions may develop. Increased blood pressure and congestive heart failure may be fatal.

Fever, sore throat, easy bruising, edema, fever and chills, leg cramps, and heart palpitations are all signs of potentially serious disorders resulting from treatment with carbamazepine. If your child experiences any of these problems, discontinue use at once and consult your pediatrician.

IMPORTANT PRECAUTIONS

Since side effects of treatment with carbamazepine (Tegretol) can be very severe, careful monitoring by your pediatrician is essential. Complete blood counts should be performed on a regular basis.

Carbamazepine is chemically related to tricyclic antidepressants such as imipramine, so it should not be given to children who are sensitive to these drugs.

Many drugs interact with carbamazepine. Carbamazepine may reduce the effectiveness of certain antibiotics such as tetracycline. Administration of carbamazepine with drugs such as cimetidine (Tagamet), erythromycin, and isoniazid may result in toxicity. The effectiveness of doxycycline, phenobarbital, phenytoin (Dilantin), theophylline, and valproic acid (Depakote) may be decreased when taken with carbamazepine.

Be certain to tell your child's pediatrician about all medications that you are giving your child, in order to properly balance drug interactions.

CEFACLOR

BRAND NAMES

Ceclor

GENERAL INFORMATION

Cefaclor is a broad-spectrum cephalosporin antibiotic prescribed to treat respiratory infections, middle ear infections, strep throat, and sinus, skin, and urinary tract infections in children. Like all cephalosporins, cefaclor is composed of penicillin molecules that have been extensively modified in the laboratory to fight different types of bacterial infections.

Cephalosporins are divided into three groups. Cefaclor is a member of the so-called second generation of cephalosporins, which are formulated to fight resistant organisms more effectively and have a broader spectrum of activity than the first generation. In addition, cefaclor can be administered less frequently than the first-generation drugs. Third-generation cephalosporins have been designed to fight off very serious, life-threatening infections.

While cefaclor and other cephalosporins are partially composed of penicillin, less than 10 percent of people allergic to penicillin are allergic to them. Cefaclor is a good-tasting antibiotic and needs to be given only twice or three times daily. On the other hand, cefaclor is more expensive than other treatment options, such as amoxicillin, with little advantage in effectiveness.

Like other antibiotics, cefaclor is effective against many susceptible *bacterial*—not viral, parasitic or fungal—infections. Your child will usually respond to treatment within several days. If he or she continues to experience fever or pain after this time, consult your pediatrician. Your child may be suffering from an infection that is resistant to cefaclor, in which case the doctor may want to see your child and/or prescribe an alternate treatment.

DOSAGE AND ADMINISTRATION

Cefaclor is available for children in suspension and capsule form. It should be administered two or three times a day. The asterisk (*) below indicates the twice daily strength. Your physician may adjust the dosage for children who fall in-between the following weights.

	125 mg suspension	187 mg suspension	250 mg suspension	375 mg suspension	250 mg capsules	500 mg capsule
12 lb	½ tsp	⅔ tsp*	—	—	—	—
22 lb	1 tsp	1 tsp*	½ tsp	½ tsp*	—	—
33 lb	1⅔ tsp	1⅔ tsp*	¾ tsp	—	—	—
44 lb	—	—	1 tsp	1 tsp*	—	—
66 lb	—	—	1–1½ tsp	1–1½ tsp*	1	—
88 lb	—	—	2 tsp	2 tsp*	2	1

SIDE EFFECTS

A common side effect of treatment with cefaclor is mild diarrhea. If this complaint becomes severe, discontinue use and consult your pediatrician.

A less common but more serious adverse reaction is enterocolitis. This condition is characterized by excessive and watery diarrhea, stomach pain, nausea, vomiting, and dehydration. If your child experiences any of these effects, discontinue use at once and consult your pediatrician.

IMPORTANT PRECAUTIONS

Cefaclor should be administered with caution to children who have experienced a sensitivity or allergic reaction to penicillin. It should not be given to children less than one month old.

CEFADROXIL

BRAND NAMES

Duricef, Ultracef

GENERAL INFORMATION

Cefadroxil is a broad-spectrum cephalosporin antibiotic prescribed to treat strep throat and skin infections, as well as respiratory, sinus, middle ear, and urinary tract infections in children. Like all cephalosporins, cefadroxil is composed of penicillin molecules that have been extensively modified in the laboratory to fight different types of bacterial infections.

Cephalosporins are divided into three groups. Cefadroxil is a member of the so-called first generation of cephalosporins, which are closest to penicillin in their action. Second-generation cephalosporins are formulated to fight resistant organisms more effectively, have a broader spectrum of activity than the first generation, and can be administered less frequently than the first-generation drugs. Third-generation cephalosporins have been designed to fight off very serious, life-threatening infections.

While cefadroxil and other cephalosporins are partially composed of penicillin, less than 10 percent of people allergic to penicillin are allergic to them. Cefadroxil is a relatively good-tasting antibiotic and needs to be given twice daily. On the other hand, cefadroxil is more expensive than other treatment options, such as amoxicillin, with little or no advantage in effectiveness.

Like other antibiotics, cefadroxil is effective against many susceptible *bacterial*—not viral, parasitic or fungal—infections. Your child will usually respond to treatment within several days. If he or she continues to experience fever or pain after this time, consult your pediatrician. Your child may be suffering from an infection that is resistant to cefadroxil, in which case the doctor may want to see your child and/or prescribe an alternate treatment.

DOSAGE AND ADMINISTRATION

Cefadroxil is available for children in suspension and capsule form. Administer as directed by your pediatrician. Your physician may adjust the dosage for children who fall in-between the following weights.

	125 mg suspension	250 mg suspension	500 mg suspension	500 mg capsules
12 lb	2/3 tsp	—	—	—
22 lb	1 1/3 tsp	—	—	—
33 lb	2 tsp	1 tsp	—	—
44 lb	—	1 1/4 tsp	2/3 tsp	—
66 lb	—	1 3/4 tsp	—	—
88 lb	—	2 tsp	1 tsp	1

SIDE EFFECTS

Common side effects of treatment with cefadroxil are mild diarrhea and yeast infections. If these complaints become severe, discontinue use and consult your pediatrician.

A less common but more serious adverse reaction is enterocolitis. This condition is characterized by excessive and watery diarrhea, stomach pain, nausea, vomiting, and dehydration. If your child experiences any of these effects, discontinue use at once and consult your pediatrician.

IMPORTANT PRECAUTIONS

Cefadroxil should be administered with caution to children who have experienced a sensitivity or allergic reaction to penicillin.

CEFIXIME

BRAND NAME

Suprax

GENERAL INFORMATION

Cefixime is a broad-spectrum cephalosporin antibiotic prescribed to treat sinus, middle ear, and respiratory infections in children. Cefixime can be especially effective against severe infections.

Cephalosporins are divided into three groups. Cefixime is a member of the so-called third generation or most powerful group of cephalosporins. These drugs have been designed to fight off very serious, even life-threatening infections, especially those that result from bacteria found in the intestine. There is considerable discussion as to whether this drug is effective against common ear and respiratory infections. It is not a drug of first choice.

Like all cephalosporins, cefixime is composed of penicillin molecules that have been extensively modified in the laboratory to fight different types of bacterial infections. Yet, while cefixime and other cephalosporins are partially composed of penicillin, less than 10 percent of people allergic to penicillin are allergic to them. Cefixime is a good-tasting antibiotic and needs to be given only once daily. On the other hand, cefixime is more expensive than other treatment options, such as amoxicillin, and may have little advantage in effectiveness.

Like other antibiotics, cefixime is effective against many susceptible *bacterial*—not viral, parasitic or fungal—infections. Your child will usually respond to treatment within several days. If he or she continues to experience fever or pain after this time, consult your pediatrician. Your child may be suffering from an infection that is resistant to cefixime, in which case the doctor may want to see your child and/or prescribe an alternate treatment.

DOSAGE AND ADMINISTRATION

Cefixime is available for children in suspension and capsule form. It should be administered once a day; a half-dose twice daily may be more effective. Doses below are for single daily doses. Your physician may adjust the dosage for children who fall in-between the following weights.

	100 mg suspension	200 tablets	400 tablets
12 lb	½ tsp	—	—
22 lb	¾ tsp	—	—
33 lb	1¼ tsp	—	—
44 lb	1⅔ tsp	—	—
66 lb	2½ tsp	1	—
88 lb	—	2	1

SIDE EFFECTS

A common side effect of treatment with cefixime is mild diarrhea. If this complaint becomes severe, discontinue use and consult your pediatrician.

A less common but more serious adverse reaction is enterocolitis. This condition is characterized by excessive and watery diarrhea, stomach pain, nausea, vomiting, and dehydration. If your child experiences any of these effects, discontinue use at once and consult your pediatrician.

IMPORTANT PRECAUTIONS

Cefixime should be administered with caution to children who have experienced a sensitivity or allergic reaction to penicillin.

CEFPROZIL

BRAND NAME

Cefzil

GENERAL INFORMATION

Cefprozil is a broad-spectrum cephalosporin antibiotic prescribed to treat respiratory infections, middle ear infections, strep throat, and sinus and skin infections in children. Like all cephalosporins, cefprozil is composed of penicillin molecules that have been extensively modified in the laboratory to fight different types of bacterial infections.

Cephalosporins are divided into three groups. Cefprozil is a member of the so-called second generation of cephalosporins, which are formulated to fight resistant organisms more effectively and have a broader spectrum of activity than the first generation. In addition, cefprozil can be administered less frequently than the first-generation drugs.

While cefprozil and other cephalosporins are partially composed of penicillin, less than 10 percent of people allergic to penicillin are allergic to them. Cefprozil is a good-tasting antibiotic and needs to be given only twice daily. On the other hand, cefprozil is more expensive than other treatment options, such as amoxicillin, with little advantage in effectiveness.

Like other antibiotics, cefprozil is effective against many susceptible *bacterial*—not viral, parasitic or fungal—infections. Your child will usually respond to treatment within several days. If he or she continues to experience fever or pain after this time, consult your pediatrician. Your child may be suffering from an infection that is resistant to cefprozil, in which case the doctor may want to see your child and/or prescribe an alternate treatment.

DOSAGE AND ADMINISTRATION

Cefprozil is available for children in suspension and capsule form. It should be administered twice a day. Your physician may adjust the dosage for children who fall in-between the following weights.

	125 mg suspension	250 mg suspension	250 mg capsules	500 mg capsules
12 lb	⅔ tsp	—	—	—
22 lb	1¼ tsp	⅔ tsp	—	—
33 lb	1¾ tsp	1 tsp	—	—
44 lb	—	1¼ tsp	1	—
66 lb	—	1¾ tsp	2	—
88 lb	—	2 tsp	2	1

SIDE EFFECTS

A common side effect of treatment with cefprozil is mild diarrhea. If this complaint becomes severe, discontinue use and consult your pediatrician.

A less common but more serious adverse reaction is enterocolitis. This condition is characterized by excessive and watery diarrhea, stomach pain, nausea, vomiting, and dehydration. If your child experiences any of these effects, discontinue use at once and consult your pediatrician.

IMPORTANT PRECAUTIONS

Cefprozil should be administered with caution to children who have experienced a sensitivity or allergic reaction to penicillin. It should not be given to children less than one month old.

CEPHALEXIN

BRAND NAME

Keflex

GENERAL INFORMATION

Cephalexin is a broad-spectrum cephalosporin antibiotic prescribed to treat strep throat and urinary tract infections, as well as skin, respiratory, and middle ear infections in children. Like all cephalosporins, cephalexin is composed of penicillin molecules that have been extensively modified in the laboratory to fight different types of bacterial infections.

Cephalosporins are divided into three groups. Cephalexin is a member of the so-called first generation of cephalosporins, which are closest to penicillin in their action.

While cephalexin and other cephalosporins are partially composed of penicillin, less than 10 percent of people allergic to penicillin are allergic to them. Cephalexin is a relatively good-tasting antibiotic but needs to be given four times daily. On the other hand, cephalexin is more expensive than other treatment options, such as amoxicillin, with little advantage in effectiveness.

Like other antibiotics, cephalexin is effective against many susceptible *bacterial*—not viral, parasitic or fungal—infections. Your child will usually respond to treatment within several days. If he or she continues to experience fever or pain after this time, consult your pediatrician. Your child may be suffering from an infection that is resistant to cephalexin, in which case the doctor may want to see your child and/or prescribe an alternate treatment.

DOSAGE AND ADMINISTRATION

Cephalexin is available for children in suspension, tablet, and capsule form. There is a wide dosage range for cephalexin. The dosage chosen, 23 mg per pound, is at the top of the dosage list. A dose 25 percent greater or 35 percent lower is within range. Cephalexin is usually given four times a day. Three doses a day are acceptable but less common. (You may calculate the dose with simple mathematics.) Your physician may adjust the dosage for children who fall in-between the following weights.

	125 mg suspension	250 mg suspension	250 mg tablets/ capsules	500 mg tablets/ capsules
12 lb	½ tsp	—	—	—
22 lb	1 tsp	—	—	—
33 lb	1½ tsp	¾ tsp	—	—
44 lb	—	1 tsp	1	—
66 lb	—	1¼ tsp	1	—
88 lb	—	1⅔–2	2	1

SIDE EFFECTS

Common side effects of treatment with cephalexin are mild diarrhea, stomachache, nausea, and vomiting. If these complaints become severe, discontinue use and consult your pediatrician.

A less common but more serious adverse reaction is enterocolitis. This condition is characterized by excessive and watery diarrhea, stomach pain, nausea, vomiting, and dehydration. If your child experiences any of these effects, discontinue use at once and consult your pediatrician.

IMPORTANT PRECAUTIONS

Cephalexin should be administered with caution to children who have experienced a sensitivity or allergic reaction to penicillin. It should not be given to children less than one month old.

CEPHRADINE

BRAND NAME

Velosef

GENERAL INFORMATION

Cephradine is a broad-spectrum cephalosporin antibiotic prescribed to treat strep throat and skin infections, as well as respiratory, sinus, middle ear, and urinary tract infections in children. Like all cephalosporins, cephradine is composed of penicillin molecules that have been extensively modified in the laboratory to fight different types of bacterial infections.

Cephalosporins are divided into three groups. Cephradine is a member of the so-called first generation of cephalosporins, which are closest to penicillin in their action.

While cephradine and other cephalosporins are partially composed of penicillin, less than 10 percent of people allergic to penicillin are allergic to them. Cephradine is a relatively good-tasting antibiotic and needs to be given only once or twice daily. On the other hand, cephradine is more expensive than other treatment options, such as amoxicillin, with little advantage in effectiveness.

Like other antibiotics, cephradine is effective against many susceptible *bacterial*—not viral, parasitic or fungal—infections. Your child will usually respond to treatment within several days. If he or she continues to experience fever or pain after this time, consult your pediatrician. Your child may be suffering from an infection that is resistant to cephradine, in which case the doctor may want to see your child and/or prescribe an alternate treatment.

DOSAGE AND ADMINISTRATION

Cephradine is available for children in suspension, tablet, and capsule form. There is a wide dosage range for cephradine. The dosage chosen, 22 mg per pound, is at the top of the dosage list. A dose 35 percent lower is within range. Cephradine is usually given four times a day. Two or three doses a day are acceptable but less common. (You may calculate the dose with simple mathematics.) Your physician may adjust the dosage for children who fall in-between the weights listed in the chart below.

	125 mg suspension	250 mg suspension	250 mg tablets/ capsules	500 mg tablets/ capsules
12 lb	½ tsp	—	—	—
22 lb	1 tsp	—	—	—
33 lb	1½ tsp	¾ tsp	—	—
44 lb	—	1 tsp	1	—
66 lb	—	1½ tsp	—	—
88 lb	—	2 tsp	2	1

SIDE EFFECTS

Common side effects of treatment with cephradine are mild diarrhea, stomachache, nausea, and vomiting. If these complaints become severe, discontinue use and consult your pediatrician.

A less common but more serious adverse reaction is enterocolitis. This condition is characterized by excessive and watery diarrhea, stomach pain, nausea, vomiting, and dehydration. If your child experiences any of these effects, discontinue use at once and consult your pediatrician.

IMPORTANT PRECAUTIONS

Cephradine should be administered with caution to children who have experienced a sensitivity or allergic reaction to penicillin. It should not be given to children less than nine months old, and should be used with caution in children who have kidney disease.

CHLORAL HYDRATE

BRAND NAMES

Aquachloral, Noctec

GENERAL INFORMATION

Chloral hydrate is prescribed to sedate children before potentially disturbing medical procedures, such as an EEG (brain wave test) or MRI. It is a very old drug with a long history of safety.

DOSAGE AND ADMINISTRATION

Chloral hydrate has a taste and odor that many children find unpleasant, and so is best administered in a manner that minimizes these effects. Refrigeration of the syrup is recommended, to downplay the taste and make it easier for your child to swallow. Mixing with fruit juice or ginger ale may help hide the taste and odor of the medication.

Chloral hydrate is available for children in syrup and suppository form. The oral and rectal dosages are the same. Doses given here are for use for sedation prior to a procedure. Medication is given one-half to one hour before the procedure. Higher doses produce more sedation and are generally more effective. A dose of 75 percent of the maximum dose is most commonly used. Your physician may adjust the dosage for children who fall in-between the following weights.

	250 mg/tsp syrup	500 mg/tsp syrup	324 mg suppository**	500 mg suppository**
12 lb	½–2 tsp*	¼–1 tsp*	1*	—
22 lb	1–4 tsp	½–2 tsp	1–3	—
33 lb	1½–6 tsp	¾–3 tsp	1–4	1–3
44 lb	—	1–4 tsp	2–6	1–4
66 lb	—	1½–4	—	1–4
88 lb	—	2–4 tsp	—	1–4

*Use of chloral hydrate on a child of this size should be done only under close medical supervision with proper monitoring by professionals experienced in its use.

**Do not cut suppositories into fractions. Medication may not be evenly distributed throughout the suppository.

SIDE EFFECTS

Stomach upset, nausea, and vomiting occur in some children who are given chloral hydrate. If one or more of these complaints become severe, consult your pediatrician.

Less frequent but more serious adverse reactions include confusion, dizziness, lightheadedness, and diarrhea. Yet these side effects are rare with the single dose that constitutes the primary use of chloral hydrate.

IMPORTANT PRECAUTIONS

Dosages of chloral hydrate should be reduced in children who have severe liver or kidney disease.

CIMETIDINE

BRAND NAME

Tagamet

GENERAL INFORMATION

Cimetidine is prescribed for the treatment of peptic ulcers and related disorders in children. This drug is a histamine receptor antagonist that works by inhibiting the actions of the chemical signals that cause gastric secretions, and is especially useful in treating reflux esophagitis (the backflow of stomach acids into the esophagus) and ulcers.

Cimetidine is usually administered for six months to a year at most. The safety and effectiveness of longer periods of therapy have not been established.

Because it has a number of potential side effects and drug interactions, cimetidine is prescribed with caution for children. In time, its chemical cousin ranitidine—which in studies thus far has demonstrated fewer side effects and drug interactions—may prove to be a favorable alternative to cimetidine.

DOSAGE AND ADMINISTRATION

Cimetidine should be taken with meals (or directly following them) and at bedtime for maximum effect.

Recommended dosages of cimetidine will depend on the nature of your child's condition. Cimetidine is usually given every six hours. Doses may be administered three to four times a day if given for a long term.

Cimetidine is available for children in syrup or tablet

form. Your physician may adjust the dosage for children who fall in-between the following weights.

	300 mg/tsp syrup	200 mg tablets	300 mg tablets	400 mg tablets
12 lb	0.25–0.5 cc*	—	—	—
22 lb	0.85–1.7 cc*	—	—	—
33 lb	¼–½ tsp	—	—	—
44 lb	⅓–⅔ tsp	—	—	—
66 lb	½–1 tsp	1–1½	½–1	—
88 lb	⅔–1⅓ tsp	1–2	1	½–1

*Dose is measured in a small syringe, usually a 1cc syringe. Note that dosage under one year of age is half the dose for greater than one year of age.

SIDE EFFECTS

The most common side effects of treatment with cimetidine (Tagamet) are diarrhea, dizziness, headache, muscle aches, and skin rashes. If one or more of these complaints become severe, discontinue use and consult your pediatrician.

A serious side effect of high doses of cimetidine is confusion. Less common adverse reactions are fever and irregular heartbeat, although studies have not definitively linked these to cimetidine. The drug has been associated with a decrease in white blood cells that fight infection (neutropenia).

If your child experiences any of these effects, discontinue use at once and consult your pediatrician. Most side effects of treatment with cimetidine are reversible and clear up several days after therapy is discontinued.

IMPORTANT PRECAUTIONS

Cimetidine (Tagamet) is a powerful drug, and is prescribed with caution in children.

Many drugs interact with cimetidine. Antacids may reduce the effectiveness of cimetidine (although, when they are taken at least one hour apart, this effect may be diminished). Administration of cimetidine with drugs such as carbamazepine, phenobarbital, phenytoin (Dilantin), and theophylline may result in toxicity.

Be certain to tell your child's pediatrician about all medications (especially daily medications) that you are giving your child, in order to properly balance drug interactions.

CLARITHROMYCIN

BRAND NAME

Biaxin

GENERAL INFORMATION

Clarithromycin is a relatively new antibiotic prescribed to treat respiratory tract and skin infections in children. Chemically related to erythromycin, clarithromycin works by preventing the growth and reproduction of susceptible bacteria. Respiratory tract infections that may respond to treatment with clarithromycin include bronchitis, strep throat, tonsillitis, sinusitis, and pneumonia.

Like other antibiotics, clarithromycin is effective against only susceptible *bacterial*—not viral, parasitic or fungal—infections. Your child will usually respond to treatment in two to five days. If he or she continues to experience fever or pain after this time, consult your pediatrician. Your child may be suffering from an infection that is resistant to clarithromycin, in which case the doctor may prescribe an alternate treatment.

DOSAGE AND ADMINISTRATION

Clarithromycin is available for children in tablet or suspension form. The suspension must *not* be refrigerated and must be thoroughly shaken before use. Many children find the suspension gritty, and it often leaves a bitter aftertaste. This can be helped by mixing the medication with chocolate ice cream and/or following the dose immediately with orange juice or cola.

Clarithromycin is administered two times a day. Your physician may adjust the dosage for children who fall in-between the following weights.

	125 mg suspension	250 mg suspension	250 mg tablets	500 mg tablets
12 lb	⅓ tsp	—	—	—
22 lb	⅔ tsp	—	—	—
33 lb	1 tsp	—	—	—
44 lb	—	⅔ tsp	—	—
66 lb	—	1 tsp	1	—
88 lb	—	1¼–2 tsp	1–2	1

SIDE EFFECTS

The most common side effect of treatment with clarithromycin is a headache. If the headache becomes severe, discontinue use and consult your pediatrician.

Less common adverse reactions include stomach discomfort, diarrhea, and nausea. If your child experiences any of these effects, discontinue use at once and consult your pediatrician.

IMPORTANT PRECAUTIONS

Clarithromycin is not an appropriate medication for a child who is sensitive or allergic to erythromycin.

For treatment with clarithromycin to be effective—and to prevent infection from recurring—it's important to follow the entire course of medication prescribed by your pediatrician, even after your child's symptoms have diminished or disappeared.

Drugs including carbamazepine (Tegretol) and theophylline are known to interact with clarithromycin. Use of clarithromycin with any of the nondrowsy antihistamines (such as Seldane, Claritin, or Hismanil) requires careful consultation with your pediatrician. Be certain to tell your child's pediatrician about all medications that you are giving your child, in order to properly balance drug interactions.

CLINDAMYCIN

BRAND NAME

Cleocin

GENERAL INFORMATION

Clindamycin is an antibiotic prescribed to treat susceptible bacterial infections in children. Clindamycin is useful in treating infections that are resistant to the penicillins and erythromycins, as well as in managing infections in children who cannot tolerate those drugs. In fact, clindamycin is the drug of choice, along with metronidazole, in serious infections caused by the most drug-resistant bacteria. These include certain abdominal and lung infections.

Clindamycin, like other antibiotics, is only effective against susceptible *bacterial*—not viral, parasitic, or fungal—infections. Your child will usually show signs of improvement following three to five days of treatment. Notify your pediatrician if toxic symptoms or discomfort persist after this time; your child may be suffering from an infection that is resistant to clindamycin, and may require an alternate treatment.

DOSAGE AND ADMINISTRATION

Clindamycin is available for children in oral liquid, capsule, and topical solution or gel form. It should be administered three or four times a day for at least ten days, with total daily dosage depending on the severity of the infection. Your physician may adjust the dosage for children who fall in-between the following weights.

	75 mg/tsp oral liquid	75 mg capsules	150 mg capsules	300 mg capsules	Topical solution or gel
12 lb	1/3–1/2 tsp*	—	—	—	—
22 lb	2/3–1 tsp.	—	—	—	—
33 lb	1–1 1/2 tsp	—	—	—	—
44 lb	1 1/3–2 tsp	—	—	—	—
66 lb	2–3 tsp	2–3	1	—	—
88 lb	2 2/3–4 tsp	3–4	2	1	twice daily

*Amounts are based on dosing 4 times daily.

SIDE EFFECTS

A common adverse effect of treatment with clindamycin is diarrhea. Medication should be discontinued, after which diarrhea normally ceases in four to fourteen days.

Nausea, vomiting, and hypersensitive reactions such as itching and rashes have also been reported. If one or more of these complaints become severe, discontinue use and consult your pediatrician.

A rare but serious side effect is that life-threatening antibiotic-related colitis may develop during or up to four weeks after treatment with clindamycin. This colitis is characterized by watery diarrhea, abdominal cramps, blood in the stools, and fever. If your child experiences any of these symptoms, discontinue use at once and consult your pediatrician. Prompt treatment is necessary to eradicate this problem.

IMPORTANT PRECAUTIONS

Clindamycin is a powerful drug, and because of its potential for serious adverse side effects should be prescribed only when clearly necessary.

For treatment with clindamycin to be effective—and to prevent infection from recurring—it's important to follow the entire course of medication prescribed by your pediatrician, even after your child's symptoms have diminished or disappeared.

Be certain to tell your child's pediatrician about all medications that you are giving your child, in order to properly balance drug interactions.

CLOBETASOL PROPIONATE

See Corticosteroids, Topical

CODEINE

GENERAL INFORMATION

Codeine is a narcotic drug prescribed to relieve mild to moderate pain and to treat coughs in children. Codeine can ease the pain following surgery or a broken bone, and it suppresses the cough reflex. Codeine is very effective when administered orally.

	10 mg/tsp codeine with dextromethorphan (for cough)	12.5 mg Elixir with 120 mg acetaminophen	7.5 mg codeine with 300 mg acetaminophen tablets	15 mg codeine with 300 mg acetaminophen tablets
12 lb	Not recommended	1/4–1/2 tsp*	—	—
22 lb	Questionable	1/3–3/4 tsp*	—	—
33 lb	1/4–1/2 tsp	2/3–1 1/4 tsp*	—	—
44 lb	1/2–3/4 tsp	3/4–1 1/2 tsp*	—	—
66 lb	3/4–1 1/4 tsp	1 1/4–2 1/2 tsp*	—	—
88 lb	1–1 1/2 tsp	1 2/3–3 1/4 tsp	2	2

*If given at the lower dose, a half-dose of acetaminophen should be given as well.

DOSAGE AND ADMINISTRATION

Codeine is almost always, because of narcotic laws, dispensed with another substance, either a cough remedy or acetaminophen. Codeine is given every four hours only as needed.

Codeine is available for children in liquid or tablet form. Your physician may adjust the dosage for children who fall in-between the weights shown on page 101.

SIDE EFFECTS

The most common side effect of treatment with codeine is dizziness. Occasionally, constipation occurs as well. If complaints become severe, discontinue use and consult your pediatrician.

Less common adverse reactions include nausea, vomiting, and drowsiness. If your child experiences any of these effects, discontinue use at once and consult your pediatrician.

IMPORTANT PRECAUTIONS

Codeine is a powerful medication and should be administered with care. Large doses of codeine can lead to respiratory depression, while long-term use of codeine causes physical dependence.

CORTICOSTEROIDS, TOPICAL

GENERAL INFORMATION

Topical corticosteroids are preparations that are used to suppress the symptoms of eczema and allergic dermatitis in children. These skin rashes are characterized by itchy red patches that may crust, scale, blister, and ooze. We do not know what causes eczema (which is also known as atopic dermatitis), although it seems to run in families. Allergic dermatitis may be caused by contact with substances such as poison ivy, oak, or sumac, nickel and other metals, chemicals in sunscreens, and topically applied drugs. It can also be caused by food allergies.

Corticosteroids work by suppressing the body's allergic response in the area treated, temporarily easing the intense itching and inflammation associated with rashes. While these medications cannot cure skin problems, their action is important both for your child's comfort and also to ward off scratching and further irritation of the skin that can lead to secondary infections.

When an allergic rash is chronic, severe, or widespread, it is important for you and your pediatrician to discover the underlying cause of the problem and eliminate it. Careful observation and a logical approach to problem-solving can help you find the answer. In the meantime, additional treatments of dermatitis include the application of lubricants and low-allergy moisturizers (such as Eucerin or Moisturelle) and oral antihistamines to reduce itching and allow your child to get a good night's sleep.

Topical corticosteroids come in two forms: hydrocortisones and halogenated corticosteroids. In the majority of circumstances, over-the-counter hydrocortisone in ½ percent strength for infants and 1 percent strength for children is sufficient. Children's skin is thinner than adults', and a less potent cream is often just as effective as a higher potency cream in an adult with the same condition. But when over-the-counter preparations cannot penetrate skin that has been thickened by chronic inflammation, more powerful prescription hydrocortisones or halogenated corticosteroids are indicated. These medications, even though applied less frequently, may cause greater side effects.

DOSAGE AND ADMINISTRATION

Topical corticosteroids should be applied exactly as directed by your pediatrician. In general, they should be used sparingly. A thin film is sufficient, and treated skin should ideally be left exposed to the air, or at most, loosely covered. Never cover with tight bandages unless specifically directed by your doctor.

SIDE EFFECTS

Side effects of treatment with topical corticosteroids are uncommon. However, chronic use of corticosteroids may result in *a serious side effect* that leaves skin thin and less resistant to injury. On rare occasions, too much of a high strength corticosteroid is spread over a large percentage of the body and is absorbed into the bloodstream. This may lead to adverse reactions such as weight gain. *A rare but potentially very serious complication* of treatment with topical corticosteroids over large areas of the body is Cushing's syndrome; this is a serious disease characterized by depression, mood swings, high blood pressure, insomnia, water retention, weight gain, round face, and muscle weakness. If your child experiences any of these effects, discontinue use at once and consult your pediatrician.

IMPORTANT PRECAUTIONS

In choosing a topical corticosteroid, choose the weakest strength that will do the job. The weaker the corticosteroid, the fewer the side effects.

There is a significant difference between brand name and generic forms of topical corticosteroids. While all of the preparations contain the same amount of active medication, many generic creams are made with inexpensive "base creams," the inactive ingredients that carry the active ingredients. If they are poorly or cheaply made, they may not let the active ingredient come in contact with the skin properly. If a generic cream is not effective, try the brand name cream of the same strength before moving on to a more powerful (and expensive) cream.

ABOUT THE CHART

Topical corticosteroids are divided into four groups, some with subgroups. Low-potency creams (which include the over-the-counter medications) are divided into Groups 7 and 6. Intermediate-potency creams (Groups 5 and 4) and high-potency creams (Groups 3 and 2) account for most of the creams sold by prescription. Ultrahigh potency creams (Group 1) are reserved for very special situations. High potency and ultrahigh potency creams should be used on children only in the most unusual circumstances and under the close supervision of a dermatologist.

Consult your pediatrician or dermatologist about which form of a preparation should be used. Creams, lotions, ointments, gels, and solutions are available, and one form may work better in a particular situation. However, the effects of any preparation in a group, when used appropriately, should be very similar.

The groupings below organize topical corticosteroids into equivalent groups. Some of the preparations may also be found in the individual profile sections. The same generic and brand names may recur in different groups, as corticosteroids can be formulated to be more or less potent. This means that, regardless of the percentage you see to the right of each drug, Group 7 corticosteroids are always weaker than those in Group 6; Group 6 corticosteroids are always weaker than those in Group 5, and so on. Brand names are listed in parentheses.

LOW POTENCY

Group 7

Dexamethasone (Hexadrol)	0.1% cream, gel
Dexamethasone	0.1% gel
Dexamethasone phosphate	0.1% gel
Hydrocortisone base or acetate (CaldeCORT or Cortaid)	0.25-2.5% lotion, cream, ointment
Methylprednisone acetate	0.25%-1% ointment

Group 6

Aclometasone dipropionate (Aclovate)	0.05% cream, ointment
Desonide (Tridesilon)	0.05% cream, ointment
Fluocinolone acetonide (Fluonid)	0.1% solution
Fluocinolone acetonide (Synalar)	0.01% cream

INTERMEDIATE POTENCY

Group 5

Betamethasone dipropionate (Diprosone)	0.05% lotion
Betamethasone valerate (Valisone)	0.1% lotion, cream, ointment
Fluocinolone acetonide (Synalar)	0.025% cream, ointment
Hydrocortisone valerate (Westcort)	0.2% cream, ointment
Triamcinolone acetonide (Kenalog, Aristocort, and others)	0.1% cream, ointment

Group 4

Desoximetasone (Topicort)	0.05% gel
Flurandrenolide (Cordran)	0.05% cream, ointment, lotion

HIGH POTENCY (RARELY NECESSARY IN CHILDREN)

Group 3

Betamethasone dipropionate (Diprosone)	0.05% cream, ointment, lotion
Diflorasone diacetate (Florone)	0.05% cream, ointment
Triamcinolone acetonide (Kenalog, Aristocort, and others)	0.5% cream, ointment

Group 2

Amcinonide (Cyclocort)	0.1% ointment
Betamethasone dipropionate (Diprosone)	0.05% cream
Desoximetasone (Topicort)	0.25% cream, ointment
Fluocinonide (Lidex)	0.05% cream, ointment, solution
Halcinomide (Halog)	0.1% cream, ointment, lotion

ULTRAHIGH POTENCY (USE IN CHILDREN ONLY WITH EXTREME CAUTION)

Group 1	
Betamethasone dipropionate (augmented)	0.05% cream, ointment
Clobetasol propionate	0.05% cream, ointment
Diflorasone diacetate (Florone)	0.05% ointment

CROMOLYN

BRAND NAMES

Intal, Nasalcrom

GENERAL INFORMATION

Cromolyn sodium is prescribed to manage the symptoms of asthma. One of the safest and most effective preventive medications for asthma in children, cromolyn works by stabilizing and preventing the release of inflammatory substances (especially histamine) from mast cells. When taken over time, cromolyn controls asthmatic symptoms triggered by allergies, cold air, and exercise. It can also be taken shortly before exercise to prevent exercise-induced asthma attacks from occurring.

Cromolyn is usually administered for two to three weeks before taking effect. Although this drug is more expensive than inhaled corticosteroids (such as beclomethasone and flunisolide), cromolyn is generally considered much safer and has been associated with far fewer side effects.

If the initial period of cromolyn therapy proves helpful, your pediatrician will most likely prescribe an individualized program of various asthma medications (such as cromolyn, bronchodilators, and inhaled corticosteroids) to maximize the benefits and minimize potential side effects for your child.

DOSAGE AND ADMINISTRATION

Cromolyn is inhaled into the lungs either through a metered-dose inhaler (MDI) or through a nebulizer. Proper use of the MDI by the use of spacer devices is essential to its effectiveness in young children.

Nebulizers are an easier way to deliver medication to small children. In this method medication is placed in a small canister attached to a face mask and then nebulized into a fine mist, which can be easily inhaled.

For the control of chronic asthma, cromolyn is initially administered three or four times daily at regular intervals during waking hours. It has been very effective in children, but is often not as effective once the child reaches adolescence.

To prevent asthma attacks that are triggered by exercise or cold air, two puffs or one ampule should be inhaled approximately 15 minutes before exposure to the irritant. The dosage does not vary with weight.

SIDE EFFECTS

Minor complaints are occasional coughing or sore throat. Based on extensive testing, cromolyn appears to be a very safe drug.

Serious adverse effects of cromolyn, such as hives and gastroenteritis, are rare, but if your child experiences one of these problems, discontinue use of cromolyn and consult your pediatrician.

IMPORTANT PRECAUTIONS

Cromolyn is a preventive medication and is not appropriate for the treatment of asthma attacks; your child will require a separate bronchodilator medication (such as albuterol) for this purpose.

Because cromolyn is a preventive, anti-inflammatory medication, results may not be evident for two to three weeks after treatment has begun. Nevertheless, in order for cromolyn to be effective, doses should be continued on a regular basis as prescribed by your pediatrician.

CYPROHEPTADINE

BRAND NAME

Periactin

GENERAL INFORMATION

Cyproheptadine is a mild oral antihistamine prescribed to treat contact irritant dermatitis and allergic reactions such as hives in children. Antihistamines work by blocking the action of histamine released from specialized allergy cells called mast cells. Histamine is the substance that most commonly causes hives, itching, and inflammation, and reactions to histamine lead to difficult breathing due to narrowing and inflammation of the airways and increased mucous secretion. Cyproheptadine has other actions against serotonin, a substance used in the transmission of signals between certain nerve cells; it is the only antihistamine to have this effect and its value is unknown.

Antihistamines including cyproheptadine can also control sensitive or allergic reactions when your child's skin comes into contact with other potential irritants, such as harsh chemicals in detergents or nickel in jewelry. Cyproheptadine may be prescribed when your child experiences penicillin sensitivity or has an allergic reaction to certain foods. It may also soothe the itch of a severe case of chicken pox.

DOSAGE AND ADMINISTRATION

Cyproheptadine works best on an empty stomach. It is not recommended for children who are under six months of age or weigh less than fourteen pounds.

Cyproheptadine is available for children in syrup or tablet

form, and should be administered every eight to twelve hours. Dosages given here are for every eight hours. If the dosages are to be given every twelve hours, give 1½ times the amount recommended here. Your physician may adjust the dosage for children who fall in-between the following weights.

	2mg/tsp syrup	4mg tablets
12 lb.	Contraindicated	—
22 lb	⅓–⅔ tsp	—
33 lb	⅔–1¼ tsp	—
44 lb	¾–1⅔ tsp	—
66 lb	1¼–2½ tsp	1
88 lb	1⅔–2⅔ tsp	1 (1–2 every 12 hours)

SIDE EFFECTS

The most common side effect of treatment with cyproheptadine is drowsiness. Dizziness, fatigue, impaired coordination, and tinnitus (ringing in the ears) may also occur. If one or more of these complaints become severe, discontinue use and consult your pediatrician.

More serious side effects occur in some children, including nervousness, irritability, and insomnia. If your child experiences any of these effects, discontinue use immediately and consult your pediatrician.

IMPORTANT PRECAUTIONS

Cyproheptadine should not be used in premature or newborn infants.

Like other antihistamines, cyproheptadine may cause drowsiness and impaired coordination. Parents might therefore choose to limit children's participation in activities such as climbing or gymnastics while taking this medication.

Other drugs may interact with cyproheptadine. Be certain

to tell your child's pediatrician about all medications that you are giving your child, in order to properly balance drug interactions.

DESMOPRESSIN ACETATE

BRAND NAMES

DDAVP, Stimate

GENERAL INFORMATION

Desmopressin acetate is a synthetic antidiuretic hormone that causes the kidneys to suppress urine production and is prescribed to assist with bedwetting in children. Desmopressin acetate is also prescribed to manage frequent urination in children who have diabetes insipidus.

DOSAGE AND ADMINISTRATION

Desmopressin acetate is available in solution form for children over sixty-six pounds, and is administered as a nose spray. The solution should be refrigerated. Doses given here are for nighttime bedwetting. Dosages for other problems are individualized and should be fully explained by the specialist treating the problem.

	Metered dose nasal spray
12 lb	Contraindicated
22 lb	Contraindicated
33 lb	Contraindicated
44 lb	Contraindicated
66 lb	1–4 sprays divided between nostrils at bedtime (1 spray in each nostril gives nighttime dryness for the vast majority of bedwetters)
88 lb	As above

SIDE EFFECTS

Side effects of treatment with desmopressin acetate are uncommon.

Adverse reactions can occur when large doses of desmopressin acetate are taken, including headaches, nausea, and a slight increase in blood pressure. In rare cases, nasal congestion and mild stomach cramps occur. If your child experiences any of these effects, discontinue use and consult your pediatrician. Reducing the dosage generally corrects problems.

IMPORTANT PRECAUTIONS

Desmopressin acetate is for nasal use only. The medication is ineffective orally.

It is important to discuss your child's fluid intake with your pediatrician. Excessive fluid intake during treatment with desmopressin acetate may result in seizures.

Desmopressin acetate should be used with caution in children who suffer from seizure disorders.

Since this medication may lead to a slight increase in blood pressure, it should also be used with caution in children who have high blood pressure or heart disease.

DESONIDE

See Corticosteroids, Topical

DESOXIMETASONE

See Corticosteroids, Topical

DEXAMETHASONE

See Corticosteroids, Topical

DEXAMETHASONE PHOSPHATE

See Corticosteroids, Topical

DEXTROAMPHETAMINE

BRAND NAME

Dexedrine

GENERAL INFORMATION

Dextroamphetamine is a stimulant prescribed to treat the behavior syndromes in children known as attention deficit hyperactivity disorder (ADHD) and attention deficit disorder (ADD). Although a stimulant, dextroamphetamine calms the hyperactive child. It is often a useful alternative to the more widely prescribed methylphenidate (Ritalin). Management of attention deficit hyperactivity disorders should also include a complete program of psychological, social, and educational treatment.

DOSAGE AND ADMINISTRATION

Dextroamphetamine is available for children in tablet and sustained-release capsule form. Initial doses can be gradually increased until behavior is effectively controlled.

The physician individualizes the dosage for each child. Higher doses are required for children with ADHD than those with ADD. Different forms may be mixed. For example, sustained-release preparations may be used during the school day, and short-acting forms after school. Children who have difficulty sleeping may benefit from an additional dose at bedtime.

As a general rule of thumb, the sustained-release capsules should be equivalent to two tablets given in sequence. For example, 1 sustained-release 10 mg capsule is equivalent to 2 5 mg tablets given three to four hours apart and should last six to eight hours. The maximum daily dosage is 40 mg.

	5 mg tablets	10 mg tablets	5 mg sustained-release	10 mg sustained-release	15 mg sustained-release
3–5 years	Begin with 2.5 mg in the morning and increase by 2.5 mg weekly until adequate control is achieved. Doses in the morning and at noon are conventional. Doses after school and in the evening are used, but not in all cases.				
6 years and older	Begin with 5 mg in the morning and increase by 5 mg weekly until adequate control is achieved. Doses in the morning and at noon are conventional. Doses after school are often used to aid with homework. Evening doses are increasingly used.				

SIDE EFFECTS

Dextroamphetamine, like all amphetamines, *has many potential side effects.* These include nervousness, restlessness, insomnia, tremors, heart problems (such as high blood pressure), dizziness, nausea, constipation, and diarrhea. At high dosages, irritability and aggressiveness may occur. If one or more of these complaints become severe, discontinue use and consult your pediatrician.

Less frequent but more serious adverse reactions include anorexia and growth retardation in children. Central nervous system reactions occur on rare occasions, while depression and psychoses have followed prolonged use of large doses. Children on stimulants may develop a nervous tic, although this usually disappears if the drug is discontinued. If your child experiences any of these effects, discontinue use at once and consult your pediatrician.

IMPORTANT PRECAUTIONS

Side effects of treatment with dextroamphetamine may be minimized by using the lowest possible effective dosage.

Children who require long-term therapy with dextroamphetamine should be monitored for potential growth problems.

In general, amphetamines are not recommended for the treatment of children who have heart or thyroid problems.

Dextroamphetamine may interact with other drugs, so be certain to tell your child's pediatrician about all medications that you are giving your child.

DICLOXACILLIN

BRAND NAMES

Dynapen, Pathocil, Veracillin

GENERAL INFORMATION

Dicloxacillin is a penicillin antibiotic prescribed to treat bacterial infections in children. It is often an effective treatment for staphylococcal infections of the skin and respiratory tract. Yet while dicloxacillin can be very effective against staphylococcal infections, it is not effective against many infections such as strep throats, that respond well to treatment with penicillin or amoxicillin.

Dicloxacillin, like other antibiotics, is only effective against susceptible *bacterial*—not viral, parasitic, or fungal—infections. Your child will usually show signs of improvement within several days. If toxic symptoms or discomfort continue after this time, consult your pediatrician. Your child may be suffering from an infection that is resistant to dicloxacillin, and your doctor may prescribe an alternate treatment.

DOSAGE AND ADMINISTRATION

Dicloxacillin should be given to children one hour before or two hours after meals.

Dicloxacillin is available for children in suspension and capsule form. The suspension should be refrigerated.

There is a broad range of dosage for this drug. Doses given here are mid-range. Patients who have been discharged from the hospital may receive doses that are double the maximum dosage recommended here. Doses below the minimum dose are likely to be ineffective in some cases.

Dicloxacillin should be administered four times a day for seven to fourteen days, with total daily dosage depending on the severity of the infection. Your physician may adjust the dosage for children who fall in-between the following weights, which are total recommended daily dosages.

	62.5 mg suspension	125 mg capsules	250 mg capsules	500 mg capsules
12 lb	½–1 tsp	—	—	—
22 lb	1–2 tsp	—	—	—
33 lb	1½–3 tsp	—	—	—
44 lb	2–4 tsp	1–2	—	—
66 lb	3–6 tsp	2–3	1	—
88 lb	—	—	1–2	1

SIDE EFFECTS

Dicloxacillin is generally a well-tolerated drug, but, like other penicillin-type drugs, dicloxacillin may cause hypersensitive or allergic reactions such as hives, and abdominal discomforts including diarrhea, nausea, and vomiting. If your child experiences any of these effects, discontinue use and consult your pediatrician.

IMPORTANT PRECAUTIONS

For treatment with dicloxacillin to be effective—and to prevent infection from recurring—it is important to follow the entire course of medication prescribed by your pediatrician, even after your child's symptoms have diminished or disappeared.

Dicloxacillin should not be given to children who have experienced a prior sensitivity or allergy to penicillin. It should be used with caution in children who have a history of severe allergic reactions to many substances.

DIFLORASONE DIACETATE

See Corticosteroids, Topical

DIPHENOXYLATE HYDROCHLORIDE WITH ATROPINE SULFATE

BRAND NAME

Lomotil

GENERAL INFORMATION

Diphenoxylate hydrochloride with atropine sulfate, more commonly known by the brand name Lomotil, is a combination medication prescribed to relieve diarrhea in children. The diphenoxylate in Lomotil limits peristalsis (contractions of the digestive tract), while the atropine adds a soothing sedative effect.

Lomotil has largely been replaced by loperamide, which is available over-the-counter as Imodium A-D and Pepto-Bismol for diarrhea. Loperamide is as effective as Lomotil and has fewer side effects, and in time may come to completely replace Lomotil. Naturally binding foods such as rice and bananas may also be helpful during a bout with diarrhea.

DOSAGE AND ADMINISTRATION

Lomotil is not an appropriate drug for children under the age of two.

It is important to pay strict attention to recommended dosages of Lomotil, since higher doses can lead to dependence, euphoria, or respiratory depression and coma. The pediatrician will reduce the dosage of Lomotil as soon as your child's diarrhea is under control.

Lomotil is available for children in syrup and tablet form. It is usually administered three times a day. Older children may take it up to four times daily, but it is usually unnecessary. Your physician may adjust the dosage for children who fall in-between the following weights.

	2.5 mg/5 ml syrup	2.5 mg tablets
12 lb	Not recommended for children under 2 years	
22 lb	⅔ tsp 3 times daily	—
33 lb	1 tsp 3 times daily	—
44 lb	1 tsp 3–4 times daily	—
66 lb	1 tsp 3–5 times daily	1 tablet 3–5 times daily
88 lb	1 tsp 3–5 times daily	1 tablet 3–5 times daily

SIDE EFFECTS

Treatment with Lomotil may cause mild symptoms of lightheadedness.

Infrequent but more serious adverse reactions include a distended or enlarged abdomen, intestinal obstruction, rash, drowsiness, depression, dizziness, restlessness, nausea, headache, and blurred vision. If your child experiences any of these effects, discontinue use and consult your pediatrician.

IMPORTANT PRECAUTIONS

Lomotil should be used with caution in children who have colitis or liver disease. Children who have Down's syndrome cannot tolerate and should not use this drug.

Drugs such as phenobarbital interact with Lomotil. Be certain to tell your child's pediatrician about all medications that you are giving your child, in order to properly balance drug interactions.

DOXYCYCLINE

BRAND NAMES

Doryx, Vibramycin

GENERAL INFORMATION

Doxycycline is a synthetic long-acting tetracycline antibiotic prescribed to treat a wide variety of bacterial infections in children. In some cases it may be more effective than tetracycline. Doxycycline, however, is not an appropriate medication for children under eight, since it may cause yellow staining on developing permanent teeth.

Doxycycline, like other antibiotics, is only effective against susceptible *bacterial*—not viral, parasitic, or fungal—infections. Your child will usually show signs of improvement following three to five days of treatment. If toxic symptoms or discomfort continue after this time, consult your pediatrician. Your child may be suffering from an infection that is resistant to doxycycline, and your doctor may want to prescribe an alternate treatment.

DOSAGE AND ADMINISTRATION

Doxycycline should be given with a glass of water to avoid irritating the throat or stomach.

Doxycycline is available for children in syrup or tablet form. It is usually administered twice a day, morning and evening.

	50 mg syrup	50 mg capsules/tablets	100 mg capsules/tablets
12 lb	Not recommended	Not recommended	Not recommended
22 lb	Not recommended	Not recommended	Not recommended
33 lb	Not recommended	Not recommended	Not recommended
44 lb	Not recommended	Not recommended	Not recommended
66 lb	1½ tsp	1	—
88 lb	2 tsp	2	1

SIDE EFFECTS

Doxycycline is generally a well-tolerated drug. Yet, like other tetracyclines, it may cause abdominal discomforts (including diarrhea) and nausea. However, diarrhea may be less common with doxycycline than with other tetracyclines. If one or more of these complaints become severe, discontinue use and consult your pediatrician.

Serious side effects of doxycycline include increased pressure in the central nervous system, causing vomiting and confusion. If your child experiences vomiting or confusion, discontinue use and consult your pediatrician.

IMPORTANT PRECAUTIONS

Doxycycline should not be given to children until their adult teeth have formed, around age eight. If given while permanent teeth are forming, it may cause permanent yellow staining of teeth.

The major concern with all the tetracycline-based drugs is skin rashes due to exposure to sunlight while taking them. Those taking doxycycline should avoid intense sunlight and use sunscreen, or discontinue the medication during times of exposure.

Drugs such as carbamazepine (Tegretol), phenytoin (Dilantin), and penicillin can interact with doxycycline. Be certain to tell your child's pediatrician about all medications that you are giving your child, in order to properly balance drug interactions.

ERYTHROMYCIN

BRAND NAMES

E-Mycin, E.E.S., EryPed, Ery-Tab, Erythrocin, Ilosone, Ilotyan, Pediamycin, Robimycin

GENERAL INFORMATION

Erythromycin is one of the safest antibiotics available today. It is prescribed to treat upper and lower respiratory tract infections (such as bronchitis, pneumonia, and strep throat), skin problems (such as the crusty, contagious rash impetigo), urinary tract infections, and pertussis (whooping cough) in infants and children.

Erythromycin is a good alternative for children who are sensitive or allergic to penicillin. It is most often prescribed to treat mild to moderate infections; severe bacterial infections in penicillin-sensitive children are more often treated with cephalosporins.

In recent years erythromycin has lost effectiveness against strep throats, at present being only 70 percent effective. In the near future it may be replaced by more broad-spectrum versions of the drug, such as clarithromycin and azithromycin.

Erythromycin, like other antibiotics, is effective only against susceptible *bacterial*—not viral, parasitic, or fungal—infections. Your child will usually show definite signs of improvement following two to five days of treatment. If toxic symptoms or discomfort persist, consult your pediatrician. Your child may be suffering from an infection that is resistant to erythromycin, in which case an alternate treatment may be prescribed.

DOSAGE AND ADMINISTRATION

Erythromycin comes in three forms:

- Erythromycin is the form most commonly used in pills. Since this form tends to irritate the stomach lining, it is often given as an enteric-coated pill that dissolves after it passes through the stomach. Plain erythromycin should be given with food, while the enteric-coated form is best absorbed on an empty stomach.
- Erythromycin ethylsuccinate is usually administered in liquid form and is best given with food.
- Erythromycin estolate is available in pill or liquid form, and is best absorbed on an empty stomach.

Because of the many forms and brands of erythromycin, we have divided them into suspensions and solid forms. Tablets, capsules, and chewable tablets are interchangeable. For older children, enteric-coated tablets give less stomach distress.

All doses are given in terms of every eight hours. At times, erythromycin, especially the ethylsuccinate, is recommended every six hours. Doses are adjusted accordingly by giving three-fourths of the recommended dose here. Doses are calculated at 18 mg per pound of weight. Doses 25 percent greater or lesser are in the normal dosing range.

Your physician may adjust the dosage for children who fall in-between the following weights.

	125 mg suspension	200 mg suspension	250 mg suspension	400 mg suspension	125 mg tablets	200 mg tablets	250 mg tablets	333 mg tablets
12 lb	½ tsp	⅓ tsp	—	—	—	—	—	—
22 lb	1 tsp	⅔ tsp	½ tsp	—	—	—	—	—
33 lb	1¼ tsp	¾ tsp	⅔ tsp	⅓ tsp	—	1	—	—
44 lb	—	1⅓ tsp	1 tsp	½ tsp	2	1	1	—
66 lb	—	2 tsp	1½ tsp	¾ tsp	3	2	1½	—
88 lb	—	—	2 tsp	1 tsp	—	2	1–2	1

SIDE EFFECTS

The most common side effects of treatment with erythromycin are stomach discomfort and vomiting. If these complaints become severe, discontinue use and consult your pediatrician.

Serious adverse reactions from erythromycin are rare in children. Mild allergic reactions, such as hives, have occurred on rare occasions. If your child experiences an allergic reaction to erythromycin, discontinue use and consult your pediatrician.

IMPORTANT PRECAUTIONS

For treatment with erythromicin to be effective—and to prevent infection from recurring—it's important to follow the entire course of medication prescribed by your pediatrician, even after your child's symptoms have diminished or disappeared.

Erythromycin should not be given to children who have experienced a prior sensitivity or allergy to this medication.

Parents of children with liver disease should consult a specialist before agreeing to treatment with erythromycin.

Many drugs interact with erythromycin. Erythromycin may increase the level of theophylline in children who are given this asthma medication. Administration of erythromycin with carbamazepine (Tegretol) can result in toxicity. Erythromycin may be incompatible with phenytoin (Dilantin), terfenadine, and tetracycline.

Be certain to tell your child's pediatrician about all medications that you are giving your child, in order to properly balance drug interactions.

ERYTHROMYCIN (EYE MEDICATION)

GENERAL INFORMATION

Erythromycin is an antibiotic prescribed in ointment form to treat eye infections in children. Eye problems such as conjunctivitis, or pinkeye, are irritating to children and extremely contagious, but prompt treatment will ordinarily clear them up within a day or two.

DOSAGE AND ADMINISTRATION

Erythromycin is available for children as an ointment. Apply a half-inch ribbon of ointment to the affected eye two to four times a day as directed. Pull down the lower lid and apply the ribbon to the inside of the lower lid.

SIDE EFFECTS

Side effects are uncommon, since erythromycin administered in this manner is not a systemic drug.

Very rarely, an allergic reaction to this drug can occur when given as an eye ointment.

IMPORTANT PRECAUTIONS

Erythromycin should be used with caution in children who

have demonstrated a previous sensitivity to this type of drug.

ERYTHROMYCIN ETHYLSUCCINATE AND SULFISOXAZOLE ACETYL

BRAND NAME

Pediazole

GENERAL INFORMATION

The combination of erythromycin ethylsuccinate and sulfisoxazole acetyl, commonly known as Pediazole, is prescribed for the treatment of severe middle ear infections in children. Children under two months of age cannot metabolize sulfisoxazole, and should not be given this drug.

In Pediazole, the antibiotic action of erythromycin ethylsuccinate is joined with a sulfa drug that prevents the growth of susceptible bacteria. Pediazole is a good choice for the treatment of strains of bacteria that are resistant to amoxicillin, the usual drug of choice for the treatment of ear infections.

DOSAGE AND ADMINISTRATION

Pediazole may be given with or without meals.

Pediazole is available for children in suspension form. Refrigeration of the suspension is not required, but it is recommended; the medication tastes better when refrigerated, which makes it easier for your child to swallow.

Children should be given Pediazole three to four times a day. If given three times daily, the dose should be increased by one-third. Your physician may also adjust the dosage for children who fall in-between the following weights.

	Suspension
12 lb	1/3 tsp
22 lb	2/3 tsp
33 lb	1 tsp
44 lb	1 1/4 tsp
66 lb	2 tsp
88 lb	2 tsp

SIDE EFFECTS

The side effects of Pediazole are those of its individual components, erythromycin ethylsuccinate and sulfisoxazole acetyl. The most common side effects of treatment with Pediazole are nausea, vomiting, and diarrhea. If one or more of these complaints become severe, discontinue use and consult your pediatrician.

Serious adverse reactions from the erythromycin component of Pediazole are rare. However, sulfisoxazole in Pediazole is a sulfa drug and *may provoke rare but severe reactions* including Stevens-Johnson syndrome (a skin condition that can be fatal), hepatitis, kidney problems, hypoglycemic blood disorders, and lupus.

Early signs of potentially severe adverse reactions to Pediazole include a sore throat, fever, paleness, purple spots on the skin, jaundice, and joint pain. If your child experiences any of these effects, discontinue use at once and consult your pediatrician.

Life-threatening episodes of anaphylaxis (an allergic reaction characterized by sudden respiratory distress, a drop in blood pressure, and the onset of hives) have also been reported. If your child goes into anaphylaxis, call 911 and describe your child's symptoms. Do not try to take your child to the emergency room yourself unless told to do so by emergency personnel. Tell the 911 operator that you need an ambulance immediately.

IMPORTANT PRECAUTIONS

For treatment with Pediazole to be effective—and to prevent infection from recurring—it's important to follow the entire course of medication prescribed by your pediatrician, even after your child's symptoms have diminished or disappeared.

Because it contains a sulfa-based drug, Pediazole should not be given to children under two months of age. Pediazole should not be prescribed for children who have experienced a prior sensitivity or allergy to either erythromycin ethylsuccinate or sulfisoxazole acetyl. It should be used with caution in children who have impaired liver or kidney function, a history of severe allergies, or asthma.

Children who have G6PD deficiency (mostly children of African or Mediterranean ancestry) should not be given this drug, as it may cause moderately severe anemia over very few hours.

Many drugs interact with Pediazole. Pediazole may increase the level of theophylline in children who are given this asthma medication. If may be incompatible with carbamazepine (Tegretol), phenytoin (Dilantin), terfenadine, and tetracycline. Combining Pediazole with any of the nondrowsy antihistamines, such as Seldane or Hismanol, should be done only after consultation.

Be certain to tell your child's pediatrician about all medications that you are giving your child, in order to properly balance drug interactions.

FLUNISOLIDE

BRAND NAMES

AeroBid, Nasalide

GENERAL INFORMATION

Flunisolide is a corticosteroid medication prescribed to prevent the symptoms of asthma. Because it is a preventive anti-inflammatory drug, flunisolide reduces inflammation in the lungs, which means both fewer asthmatic episodes and a reduced possibility of permanent lung damage due to asthma.

DOSAGE AND ADMINISTRATION

Flunisolide is inhaled into the lungs through metered-dose inhalers, nebulizers, or nasal spray. Breathing in medication is an effective way of getting it directly into the airways.

Metered-dose inhalers, or MDIs, can be used by children once they are ten years old. An MDI is a small hand-held device from which the appropriate dose of medication is released into the mouth as the child breathes in. Younger children can use spacer devices with MDIs.

Nebulizers are an easier way to deliver medication to small children. In this method, medication is placed in a small canister attached to a face mask and then nebulized into a fine mist, which can be easily inhaled.

Flunisolide is normally administered in one or two inhalations two times a day. The dosage does not vary with age.

SIDE EFFECTS

The most common side effects of treatment with flunisolide are dry mouth, hoarseness, and sore throat. Rinsing the mouth after using is an easy way to prevent most side effects.

Less common adverse reactions include yeast infections of the mouth or larynx, which are characterized by a persistent sensitive throat. If your child experiences one of these problems, discontinue use and consult your pediatrician. Antifungal medication may be required.

IMPORTANT PRECAUTIONS

Flunisolide is a preventive medication and is not appropriate for the treatment of asthma attacks. Your child will most likely require a separate bronchodilator medication (such as albuterol) for this purpose.

Because flunisolide is a preventive, anti-inflammatory medication, results may not be evident for one to two weeks after treatment has begun.

Only your pediatrician should make adjustments in dosage. In order for flunisolide to be effective, doses should be continued on a regular basis exactly as prescribed by your pediatrician, whether or not symptoms are present. Dosages likewise should not be increased unless your pediatrician directs you to do so.

When using both bronchodilator and flunisolide medications to control your child's asthma, the bronchodilator should be given first in order to optimize the effectiveness of flunisolide.

FLUOCINOLONE ACETONIDE

See Corticosteroids, Topical

FLUOCINONIDE

BRAND NAMES

Lidex, Topsyn

GENERAL INFORMATION

Fluocinonide is a topical anti-inflammatory corticosteroid prescribed to relieve skin rashes in children. These itchy, irritating, and often oozing rashes include eczema, contact dermatitis (a rash due to contact with irritants ranging from poison ivy to detergents used to wash clothing to nickel in jewelry), and psoriasis.

While the exact causes of most rashes remain unknown, certain children appear especially prone to developing them, probably due to genetic predisposition. Identifying and avoiding the substance or substances that trigger rashes is important, as is keeping your child's fingernails well-clipped when rashes develop.

Depending on the severity of the rash, your pediatrician will recommend an over-the-counter product such as hydrocortisone ½ or 1 percent (CaldeCORT or Cortaid), a mild prescription topical corticosteroid such as this one, or a more potent preparation such as betamethasone. (For a comprehensive discussion of topical corticosteroids, turn to page 102.)

DOSAGE AND ADMINISTRATION

Fluocinonide is available in cream, gel, and ointment form. Apply once or twice daily, as directed by your pediatrician. A thin film is sufficient, and treated skin should ideally be left exposed to the air, or, at most, loosely covered. Never cover with tight bandages except at the recommendation of a dermatologist.

SIDE EFFECTS

The most common side effect of treatment with fluocinonide is thinning of the skin, especially when it is used on sensitive areas such as the face, neck, or genitals. Use the smallest effective amount to protect the skin.

Less common adverse reactions include persistent redness or raised bumps on the skin, which may indicate skin disorders such as acne, rosacea, miliaria, and folliculitis. A rare but potentially very serious complication of treatment with topical corticosteroids over large areas of the body is Cushing's syndrome; this is a serious disease characterized by depression, mood swings, high blood pressure, insomnia, water retention, weight gain, round face, and muscle weakness. If your child experiences any of these effects, discontinue use at once and consult your pediatrician.

IMPORTANT PRECAUTIONS

While fluocinonide is very effective in relieving skin rashes, even small amounts of topical corticosteroids can be absorbed through the skin and disrupt adrenal function. This is an especially serious concern for children, since the production of growth hormones may be disrupted.

The single most important thing to remember when using fluocinonide in children is to use it for a short period of time, usually one week. Apply fluocinonide only as directed by your pediatrician, and use it sparingly. Chronic daily use should be under close medical supervision.

Fluocinonide is for external use only. Do not apply it in the sensitive area around your child's eyes.

FLUORIDE WITH VITAMINS AND MINERALS

BRAND NAMES

Luride, Poly-Vi-Flor, Tri-Vi-Flor

GENERAL INFORMATION

Dietary supplements are prescribed to ensure that your child receives the appropriate amounts of fluoride, vitamins, and minerals for optimum health. Many public water supplies contain adequate amounts of fluoride, and food is the best source of vitamins and minerals. However, if the water supply where you live does not have adequate fluoride, a fluoride supplement is a must for healthy teeth. Finicky eaters may also benefit from a dietary supplement. Check with your water supplier, dentist, or pediatrician to find out if a dietary supplement is right for your child.

DOSAGE AND ADMINISTRATION

Fluoride supplements are recommended in areas where there is little or no fluoride in the drinking water. The concentration of fluoride is given in parts per million. If there are more than 0.7 parts per million (ppm) of fluoride in your water supply, supplements are unnecessary and can even lead to tooth damage.

The first dosage given below is for areas with less than 0.3 ppm of fluoride in the water supply; the dosage in brackets [ ] is for those areas with 0.3 to 0.7 ppm of fluoride. Fluoride supplements should be given once a day.

	Luride Drops (0.5mg/1 ml)	Poly-Tri-Vi-Flor (Dose is 1.0 ml; the concentration is varied instead)	Chewable fluoride (0.5 mg)	Poly-Vi-Flor (1 mg) and other chewable tablets (1 mg)
6 months–2 years	½ ml [none]	0.25 mg concentration [do not use]	—	—
2 years	1 ml [½ ml]	.5 mg concentration [.25 mg concentration]	1 tablet [do not use]	—
≥ 3 years	2 ml [1 ml]	—	2 tablets [1 tablet]	1 [do not use]

SIDE EFFECTS

None.

IMPORTANT PRECAUTIONS

Excessive amounts of vitamins and minerals can be toxic. Excessive amounts of fluoride may cause mottling of the teeth. It is important to check with your pediatrician, dentist, or local water district to determine whether the water supply contains fluoride. Be sure to follow your pediatricians's instructions and do not exceed recommended dosage.

FLURANDRENOLIDE

See Corticosteroids, Topical

GAMMA BENZENE HEXACHLORIDE

BRAND NAMES

Kwell, Lindane

GENERAL INFORMATION

Gamma benzene hexachloride is prescribed to treat lice and scabies infestations of the skin and scalp in children. Children are in frequent physical contact with one another, so parasites such as these are very likely to pass from one child to the next. Lice are generally a more common problem than scabies.

To detect head lice, search for small white eggs or nits that look like lint or dandruff in the hair follicles at the base of your child's scalp. If you find a nit, try to remove it from the hair shaft with your fingernails. If it doesn't come off, your child probably has lice.

Scabies are more difficult to detect. Intense itching and sores that resemble boils are the signs of scabies in children. Diagnosis is made by your pediatrician from the examination of skin scrapings.

In addition to using gamma benzene hexachloride to get rid of the current infestation, you will need to take steps to prevent reinfestation. These include laundering your child's clothing, towels, and bedding in the hot water cycle; thoroughly vacuuming all carpets in your home; storing items that cannot be washed or dry-cleaned in plastic bags for two weeks. Parasites can otherwise persist in the child's environment and reinfest them.

DOSAGE AND ADMINISTRATION

Gamma benzene hexachloride is not an appropriate remedy for infants. It is available as shampoo for the treatment of lice in hairy areas and in lotion or cream form for body lice (scabies). Although gamma benzene hexachloride can be applied at seven-day intervals, a single treatment is preferable.

For Lice: For head lice, apply one ounce of the shampoo to dry hair and leave in place for six to eight minutes before thoroughly rinsing. Remove nits with a nit comb or tweezers. Repeat in seven days if lice return.

For Scabies: Apply gamma benzene hexachloride cream or lotion to the affected skin following a lukewarm bath at bedtime. Do not exceed the prescribed dose, and avoid the eyes and mucous membranes. Following an overnight application, thoroughly rinse your child's body of all traces of gamma benzene hexachloride. A single overnight application is sufficient.

SIDE EFFECTS

Common side effects include irritation of the skin, eyes, and mucous membranes, and allergic reactions. Skin irritation can occur when gamma benzene hexachloride is used too frequently over an extended period of time. If irritation becomes severe, discontinue use and consult your pediatrician.

Serious adverse reactions to gamma benzene hexachloride can occur when it is absorbed through the skin in large amounts. Toxic reactions such as seizures can result. If you suspect that your child is experiencing a toxic reaction to gamma benzene hexachloride, discontinue use and consult your pediatrician at once.

IMPORTANT PRECAUTIONS

Gamma benzene hexachloride should be used with extreme caution in young children.

Gamma benzene hexachloride is *not* for internal use. If you suspect that your child has swallowed any, call your poison control center.

Gamma benzene hexachloride should not be used on open sores or wounds.

Avoid unnecessary skin contact. Always wear rubber gloves. This is especially important if you are pregnant or nursing.

Take care that your child's eyes are protected from the shampoo. If shampoo accidentally enters eyes, immediately flush them with plenty of cold water.

Avoid inhaling all fumes of gamma benzene hexachloride.

Be careful to follow all directions. Apply in a well-ventilated room.

If your child is prone to allergic reactions of the skin, consult your pediatrician before using gamma benzene hexachloride.

GRISEOFULVIN

BRAND NAMES

Microcrystalline: Fulvicin, Grifulvin V, Grisactin
Ultracrystalline: Fulvicin P/G, Gris-PEG, Grisactin Ultra

GENERAL INFORMATION

Griseofulvin is prescribed to treat a number of fungal infections of the skin, hair, and nails. These include athlete's foot and ringworm of the body, groin, nails, and scalp. Griseofulvin comes in two forms: microcrystalline and ultracrystalline. The ultracrystalline form is smaller, is better absorbed, and requires a lower dose; otherwise they are the same drug.

Since griseofulvin is effective for only certain types of skin infections—notably those caused by epidermophyton, microsporum, and trichophyton fungi—your pediatrician or dermatologist may perform tests before treatment to determine the particular fungus responsible for your child's infection. In general, griseofulvin is prescribed for stubborn infections that defy topical treatment. Minor infections—with the exception of scalp infections, which usually require griseofulvin—are more appropriately treated with local antifungal creams. Some infections, specifically those of the nails, may require long-term treatment.

DOSAGE AND ADMINISTRATION

Griseofulvin is generally not recommended for children under the age of two. This medication should be given to your child with meals that include milk, eggs, or high-fat foods. High-fat foods enhance its absorption from the intestine.

Griseofulvin is available for children in suspension, capsule, and tablet form. The dose used here, 9 mg per pound, has recently been recommended for children because of increasing resistance to the medication. Dosages here are one-third higher than recommended in many other texts for that reason. Your physician may adjust the dosage for children who fall in-between the following weights.

	125 mg micro-size suspension	125 mg capsules	250 mg capsules/tablets	500 mg tablets	125 mg ultra-micro-size tablets*	250 mg ultra-micro-size tablets*
12 lb	Not approved for children under 2 years of age. Use under 2 years of age should be supervised by a dermatologist or physician experienced with the drug in this age group.					
22 lb	1⅔ tsp	—	—	—	—	—
33 lb	2⅓ tsp	2	1	—	1	—
44 lb	3¼ tsp	3	—	—	—	—
66 lb	5 tsp	5	2	—	2	1
88 lb	6½ tsp	6	3–4	2	3–4	2

*Dosages of ultramicrosize forms are half that of microsize forms, hence the lower dose.

SIDE EFFECTS

Common side effects of treatment with griseofulvin include headache and skin rashes. If complaints become severe, discontinue use and consult your pediatrician.

Less common serious side effects or adverse reactions are confusion, diarrhea, hives, dizziness, fatigue, insomnia, nausea, and vomiting. If your child experiences any of these effects, discontinue use and consult your pediatrician.

IMPORTANT PRECAUTIONS

For treatment with griseofulvin to be effective—and to prevent infection from recurring—it's important to follow the entire course of medication prescribed by your pediatrician, which may vary from two weeks to several months, depending on the nature of the infection.

Griseofulvin should be administered with caution to children who have a history of allergic reactions to penicillin. Since griseofulvin is derived from a species of penicillin, be certain to notify your pediatrician if your child is sensitive or allergic to penicillin.

Griseofulvin can cause skin rashes with exposure to intense sunlight. The use of sunscreens or avoidance of intense sun exposure is recommended.

GUAIFENESIN, PSEUDOEPHEDRINE, AND CODEINE

BRAND NAME

Nucofed Pediatric Expectorant

GENERAL INFORMATION

Nucofed Pediatric Expectorant is prescribed to relieve cough and cold symptoms in children. Because it contains codeine, Nucofed can be very effective in controlling coughs. However, since codeine is serious medicine for children, your pediatrician will usually recommend that you try over-the-counter products before turning to Nucofed. (For more information about cough and cold preparations, turn to page 239.)

	Syrup
12 lb	Not recommended
22 lb	¼–½ tsp every 4–6 hours
33 lb	½ tsp every 4–6 hours
44 lb	½–¾ tsp every 4–6 hours
66 lb	½–1 tsp every 4–6 hours
88 lb	1–2 tsp every 4–6 hours

DOSAGE AND ADMINISTRATION

Nucofed is not recommended for children under age one. It should be administered to children three to four times a day as needed for a one-week period. Nucofed is available in syrup form.

SIDE EFFECTS

The most common side effects of treatment with Nucofed are sleepiness, dry mouth and throat, dizziness, and constipation. If one or more of these complaints become severe, discontinue use and consult your pediatrician.

Less common serious side effects or adverse reactions include nausea, vomiting, and nervousness. If your child experiences any of these effects, discontinue use at once and consult your pediatrician.

IMPORTANT PRECAUTIONS

Nucofed Pediatric Expectorant is a powerful medication and should be administered with care. Large doses of products that contain codeine can lead to respiratory depression, while long-term use of codeine causes physical dependence.

HALCINONIDE

See Corticosteroids, Topical

HYDROCORTISONE VALERATE

See Corticosteroids, Topical

HYDROXYZINE

BRAND NAMES

Atarax, Vistaril

GENERAL INFORMATION

Hydroxyzine is an oral antihistamine prescribed to control itching due to an allergic reaction. It is used to treat hives and may help reduce the amount of scratching in children with atopic dermatitis (eczema). Hydroxyzine is especially helpful when topical products alone are insufficient to control itching and inflammation.

Antihistamines work by blocking the action of histamine released from specialized allergy cells called mast cells. Histamine is the substance that most commonly causes itching and inflammation, and reactions to histamine can lead to difficulty in breathing due to narrowing and inflammation of the airways and increased mucous secretion.

Antihistamines such as hydroxyzine can also control sensitive or allergic reactions when your child's skin comes into contact with potential irritants, such as harsh chemicals in detergents or nickel in jewelry. Hydroxyzine may be prescribed when your child experiences penicillin sensitivity or has an allergic reaction to certain foods. It may also soothe the itch of a severe case of chicken pox.

Hydroxyzine often has a calming, sedative effect upon children as well. Because it makes individuals drowsy, hydroxyzine has been used to sedate an anxious patient. However, although it is widely used for this purpose, experts question whether that use is actually appropriate.

DOSAGE AND ADMINISTRATION

Hydroxyzine is available for children in syrup and capsule form. It is given in three or four doses daily every six to eight hours, for as long as symptoms persist. The doses stated are for four doses the first day and three doses per day on subsequent days. Your physician may adjust the dosage for children who fall in-between the following weights.

	10 mg syrup	25 mg capsules	50 mg capsules
12 lb	1/4–1/3 tsp	—	—
22 lb	1/2–2/3 tsp	—	—
33 lb	3/4–1 tsp	—	—
44 lb	1–1 1/3 tsp	—	—
66 lb	1 1/2–2 tsp	—	—
88 lb	—	1–4*	1–2*

*These doses are generally 25–50 mg but may go higher, depending on symptoms and tolerance of side effects (principally drowsiness).

SIDE EFFECTS

The most common side effect from hydroxyzine is drowsiness.

Less common serious side effects or adverse reactions are dry mouth, involuntary motor activity, tremor, and convulsions. If your child experiences any of these effects, discontinue use at once and consult your pediatrician.

IMPORTANT PRECAUTIONS

Like other antihistamines, hydroxyzine may cause drowsiness and impaired coordination. Parents should therefore limit certain activities, such as climbing or gymnastics, when children are taking this medication.

Other drugs, such as phenobarbital, interact with hydroxyzine. Be certain to tell your child's pediatrician about all medications that you are giving your child, in order to properly balance drug interactions.

HYOSCYAMINE SULFATE, ATROPINE SULFATE, SCOPOLAMINE HYDROBROMIDE, AND PHENOBARBITAL

BRAND NAME

Donnatal

GENERAL INFORMATION

The drug commonly known as Donnatal is prescribed to control intestinal cramps and diarrhea in children. The ingredients hyoscyamine sulfate, atropine sulfate, scopolamine hydrobromide, and phenobarbital are combined to prevent peristalsis, or contractions of the digestive tract. One ingredient, phenobarbital, acts as a mild sedative.

Donnatal is an old remedy and contains many drugs that have only short-term effects for stomach cramps and have not been shown to be effective for diarrhea. Over-the-counter medications, such as Imodium A-D and Pepto-Bismol for diarrhea, may be equally or more effective with fewer side effects. Naturally binding foods such as rice and bananas may also be helpful during a bout with diarrhea.

DOSAGE AND ADMINISTRATION

Donnatal is available for children in elixir, tablet, and capsule form. It should be administered every four to six hours,

	Elixir	Tablets/capsules
12 lb	0.6 ml	—
22 lb	1.0 ml	—
33 lb	1.5 ml	—
44 lb	½ tsp	—
66 lb	¾ tsp	—
88 lb	1–2 tsp	1–2 tablets

but not more than four doses per day. Your physician may adjust the dosage for children who fall in-between the weights in the chart on the facing page.

SIDE EFFECTS

Common side effects of treatment with Donnatal are blurred vision, constipation, decreased sweating, drowsiness, and dry mouth. If one or more of these complaints become severe, discontinue use and consult your pediatrician.

Infrequent serious side effects or adverse reactions include difficulty swallowing, dizziness, headache, nausea, and vomiting. If your child experiences any of these effects, discontinue use at once and consult your pediatrician.

IMPORTANT PRECAUTIONS

Donnatal is for short-term use only; your pediatrician will reduce the dosage as soon as your child's diarrhea is under control.

Donnatal should be used with caution in children who have colitis, high blood pressure, kidney or liver disease.

Many drugs, including certain antihistamines and barbiturates, can interact with Donnatal. Be certain to tell your child's pediatrician about all medications that you are giving your child, in order to properly balance drug interactions.

IMIPRAMINE

BRAND NAME

Tofranil

GENERAL INFORMATION

Imipramine is a tricyclic antidepressant prescribed to control bed-wetting problems (enuresis) in children. Although imipramine is routinely and successfully used for this purpose, exactly how it works remains unclear. Imipramine is usually combined with behavioral therapies for a two- to three-month period. It is not FDA-approved for the treatment of depression in children; physicians treating depression with this drug should be specially qualified in its use in children.

DOSAGE AND ADMINISTRATION

Imipramine is not an appropriate remedy for children under six.

Imipramine is available for children over six in tablet or capsule form. The duration of treatment is two to three months. Dosage begins at 25 mg and is increased until dryness occurs or a dose of 75 mg is reached.

Imipramine is administered as one daily dose after dinner or up to one hour before bedtime. Your physician may adjust the dosage for children who fall in-between the following weights.

	25 mg tablets	50 mg tablets	75 mg tablets/ capsules
12 lb	Children under 6 should not receive drug treatment for enuresis (bed-wetting)		
22 lb			
33 lb			
44 lb	1–3	1	1
66 lb	1–3	1	1
88 lb	1–3	1	1

SIDE EFFECTS

Common adverse effects of imipramine include drowsiness, dry mouth, nausea, vomiting, blurred vision, restlessness, sleep disturbances, and mood changes. If one or more of these complaints become severe, discontinue use and consult your pediatrician.

Withdrawal reactions such as nausea, headache, and malaise may occur after long-term therapy if imipramine is discontinued too abruptly.

IMPORTANT PRECAUTIONS

Children taking imipramine should have a cardiogram, blood pressure check, and complete blood count at the start of therapy and with each increase in therapy.

High amounts of imipramine in children may cause convulsions and coma, and overdosage can be fatal. The drug should be stored in a childproof container out of reach of children and should never be referred to as "candy." Be sure to follow your pediatrician's instructions and do not exceed recommended dosage.

ISONIAZID

BRAND NAMES

INH, Isotamine, Laniazid, Nydrazid, Rifamate, Rimifon, Tubizid

GENERAL INFORMATION

Isoniazid is an antibacterial agent prescribed for the treatment of children who have been exposed to tuberculosis but who have no evidence of active disease. This means that their TB test has become positive but they have no evidence of active tuberculosis (i.e., a negative chest X ray). Active TB is quite rare among children and requires multiple drug therapy. We do not cover it in this book.

DOSAGE AND ADMINISTRATION

Isoniazid is available for children in syrup or tablet form. It is usually administered once a day, although the drug dosage can be doubled and given twice weekly after the first month in situations where it is hard to medicate children daily. Treatment is for nine months in all cases. Your physician may adjust the dosage for children who fall in-between the following weights.

	50 mg syrup*	50 mg tablet	100 mg tablet	300 mg tablet
12 lb	1 tsp	1 tablet, crushed	—	—
22 lb	2 tsp	—	1 tablet, crushed	—
33 lb	3 tsp	3 tablets, crushed	—	—
44 lb	4 tsp	—	2 tablets, crushed	—
66 lb	6 tsp	—	—	1 tablet
88 lb	—	—	—	1 tablet

*If syrup is not available, your pharmacist may be able to prepare one for you. Tablets can be crushed and mixed with applesauce.

SIDE EFFECTS

Side effects of treatment with isoniazid are uncommon.

Infrequent serious side effects or adverse reactions include confusion, muscle pain, and tingling or numbness. Rare complications of treatment with isoniazid are convulsions and peripheral neuritis (numbness and tingling due to nerve inflammation). If your child experiences any of these effects, discontinue use at once and consult your pediatrician. Problems can usually be prevented or controlled by using a low dosage.

IMPORTANT PRECAUTIONS

Isoniazid should be used with caution in children who suffer from diabetes mellitus or malnutrition. Supplementary vitamin B6 and monitoring of liver function may be necessary in children with underlying medical conditions.

Isoniazid interacts with many other drugs, including ketoconazole and phenytoin (Dilantin). Be certain to tell your child's pediatrician about all medications that you are giving your child, in order to properly balance drug interactions.

KETOCONAZOLE

BRAND NAME

Nizoral

GENERAL INFORMATION

Ketoconazole is prescribed to treat susceptible fungal infections in children, such as oral thrush (which is characterized by milky-white patches in the mouth) and candidiasis. Ketoconazole may be especially useful in coping with hard-to-treat infections that have not responded to griseofulvin.

DOSAGE AND ADMINISTRATION

Ketoconazole is not an appropriate remedy for children under two. It should be given with liquid or food to avoid stomach irritation.

Ketoconazole is available for children in suspension, tablet, and topical form. Duration of treatment depends upon the nature of the infection being treated. The dose is given once daily. Your physician may adjust the dosage for children who fall in-between the following weights.

	100 mg suspension*	200 mg tablets	Topical
12 lb	Not approved for use in children less than 2 years (may be used in this age group under special circumstances)		Apply to affected area once or twice daily.
22 lb	½–1 tsp once daily**	—	
33 lb	¾–1½ tsp**	—	
44 lb	1–2 tsp daily**	1 tablet daily	
66 lb	1½–3 tsp daily**	1–1½ tablets daily	
88 lb	—	2 tablets daily**	

*Your pharmacist must make this, according to instructions contained in the *Handbook of Extemporaneous Formulations*, published by the American Society of Hospital Pharmacists.

**May be given in half-dose twice daily.

SIDE EFFECTS

Common side effects of treatment with ketoconazole include nausea and itching. If one or more of these complaints become severe, discontinue use and consult your pediatrician.

Less common serious side effects or adverse reactions include headache, dizziness, stomach pain, constipation, diarrhea, and nervousness. *A rare but very serious adverse effect* is hepatitis, which is indicated by loss of appetite, fatigue, nausea, vomiting, dark urine, and pale stools. If your child experiences any of these effects, discontinue use at once and consult your pediatrician.

IMPORTANT PRECAUTIONS

Ketoconazole is not an appropriate medication for children under the age of two unless they have special medical problems and are under the care of specialists.

For treatment with ketoconazole to be effective—and to prevent infection from recurring—it's important to follow the entire course of medication prescribed by your pediatrician, which may vary from two weeks to several months, depending on the nature of the infection. The cure is determined when symptoms disappear and laboratory cultures are negative.

Ketoconazole interacts with many other drugs. Cimetidine (Tagamet), isoniazid, and ranitidine may decrease the metabolism of ketoconazole. Taking ketoconazole and phenytoin (Dilantin) together may alter the effect of both drugs. When ketoconazole and terfenadine or cimetidine are taken at the same time, a life-threatening irregular heartbeat may develop. Ketoconazole should not be given at the same time or should be used with caution with terfenadine and other nondrowsy antihistamines.

Be certain to tell your child's pediatrician about all medications that you are giving your child, in order to properly balance drug interactions.

LIDOCAINE

BRAND NAME

Xylocaine

GENERAL INFORMATION

Lidocaine is a local anesthetic prescribed to relieve mouth pain and irritation in children. It is used for problems such as toothaches, teething pain, sore gums, and cold sores. However, since lidocaine is a potent anesthetic, this drug should only be used after other alternatives—including ice cubes, teething biscuits, and over-the-counter remedies such as Anbesol and Orajel—have proven insufficient.

DOSAGE AND ADMINISTRATION

A 2 percent solution or gel of lidocaine is usually recommended for topical anesthesia in children. The dosage is not weight- or age-dependent. Apply to sore areas of your child's mouth with a cotton-tipped applicator. Apply the smallest effective amount as needed.

SIDE EFFECTS

Lidocaine is not irritating and rarely provokes sensitive or allergic reactions.

Large amounts of lidocaine can cause an arrhythmic heartbeat. This problem can usually be controlled by using small amounts of lidocaine only when necessary. If your child shows signs of either unusual stimulation and excitement or depression and sleepiness, discontinue use at once and consult your pediatrician.

IMPORTANT PRECAUTIONS

Do not give your child anything to eat or drink for an hour after administering lidocaine. Numbness might make it difficult for children to swallow correctly.

Only small amounts of lidocaine are necessary to relieve

your child's pain and discomfort; also keep in mind that smaller amounts are less likely to cause adverse reactions.

LORACARBEF

BRAND NAME

Lorabid

GENERAL INFORMATION

Loracarbef is a broad-spectrum cephalosporin antibiotic prescribed to treat respiratory infections, middle ear infections, strep throat, and sinus, skin, and urinary tract infections in children. Like all cephalosporins, loracarbef is composed of penicillin molecules that have been extensively modified in the laboratory to fight different types of bacterial infections.

Cephalosporins are divided into three groups. Loracarbef is a member of the so-called second generation of cephalosporins, which are formulated to fight resistant organisms more effectively and have a broader spectrum of activity than the first generation. In addition, loracarbef can be administered less frequently than the first-generation drugs. Third-generation cephalosporins have been designed to fight off very serious, life-threatening infections.

While loracarbef and other cephalosporins are partially composed of penicillin, less than 10 percent of people allergic to penicillin are allergic to them. Loracarbef is a good-tasting antibiotic and needs to be given only once or twice daily. On the other hand, loracarbef is more expensive than other treatment options, such as amoxicillin, with little advantage in effectiveness.

Like other antibiotics, loracarbef is effective against many susceptible *bacterial*—not viral, parasitic or fungal—infections. Your child will usually respond to treatment within several days. If he or she continues to experience fever or pain after this time, consult your pediatrician. Your child may be suffering from an infection that is resistant to loracarbef, in which case the doctor may want to see your child and/or prescribe an alternate treatment.

DOSAGE AND ADMINISTRATION

Loracarbef is available for children in suspension and capsule form. It should be administered twice a day. The dosage for streptococcal sore throat is one-half that stated. Your physician may adjust the dosage for children who fall in-between the following weights.

	125 mg suspension	250 mg suspension	250 mg capsules	500 mg capsules
12 lb	⅔ tsp	—	—	—
22 lb	1¼ tsp	⅔ tsp	—	—
33 lb	1⅔ tsp	1 tsp	—	—
44 lb	—	1¼	1	—
66 lb	—	1¾	2	—
88 lb	—	2	2	1

SIDE EFFECTS

A common side effect of treatment with loracarbef is mild diarrhea. If this complaint becomes severe, discontinue use and consult your pediatrician.

A less common but more serious adverse reaction is enterocolitis. This condition is characterized by excessive, watery diarrhea, stomach pain, nausea, vomiting, and dehydration. This occurs when loracarbef is used for a prolonged time, beyond the usual 10 days of therapy. If your child experiences any of these effects, discontinue use at once and consult your pediatrician.

IMPORTANT PRECAUTIONS

Loracarbef should be administered with caution to children who have experienced a sensitivity or allergic reaction to penicillin. In addition, other drugs may interact with loracarbef. Be certain to tell your child's pediatrician about all medications that you are giving your child, in order to properly balance drug interactions.

MEBENDAZOLE

BRAND NAMES

Mebendacin, Mebutar, Nemasole, Vermox

GENERAL INFORMATION

Mebendazole is an antiparasitic drug prescribed to treat hookworm, roundworm, pinworm, whipworm, and mixed worm infections in children.

DOSAGE AND ADMINISTRATION

Mebendazole is available for children in tablet form.

	100 mg chewable tablet for pinworm treatment	100 mg chewable tablet for other parasites (hookworm and roundworm)
12 lb	1 tablet, chewed, crushed with food or swallowed, repeated in 10 days. Weight or age are not a factor in dosage.	1 tablet, chewed, crushed with food or swallowed twice daily for 3 days. Weight or age are not a factor in dosage.
22 lb		
33 lb		
44 lb		
66 lb		
88 lb		

SIDE EFFECTS

There are no minor side effects. While serious side effects are extremely rare, if your child experiences any ill effects, discontinue use and consult your pediatrician.

IMPORTANT PRECAUTIONS

Mebendazole has not been extensively investigated and therefore is not recommended for children under two.

METHYLPHENIDATE

BRAND NAME

Ritalin

GENERAL INFORMATION

Methylphenidate is prescribed to treat the behavioral syndrome known as attention deficit hyperactivity disorder (ADHD) and attention deficit disorder (ADD) in children. Although methylphenidate is a mild central nervous system stimulant, it acts to calm hyperactive children.

Methylphenidate contributes to the management of overactivity and lengthens the attention spans of hyperactive children. In comparative studies, methylphenidate was shown to be a more effective treatment for ADHD than either dextroamphetamine or pemoline. Management of attention deficit hyperactivity disorders should also include a complete program of psychological, social, and educational treatment.

DOSAGE AND ADMINISTRATION

The recommended dosage schedule of methylphenidate for children is two or three times a day. A single daily dose is not an effective treatment. Doses are most often given in the morning, at noon, and after school.

The initial dosage is 5 mg. This dose can be increased at the rate of 5 mg per dose every three or four days until the condition is under control, without causing troublesome side effects. (Dosage should be reduced if your child becomes withdrawn, tearful, or suspicious.) The maximum daily dosage is 60 mg.

Methylphenidate should be administered at mealtime to avoid appetite suppression. Dosage schedules must be individualized for each child. Children who have difficulty sleeping, for example, may benefit from an additional dose at bedtime.

Doses are given for the initial dose by weight and for the amount the dose is increased each week (initial/weekly increase).

<table>
<tr><th></th><th>5 mg tablet</th><th>10 mg tablet</th><th>20 mg tablet</th><th>20 mg sustained release tablet</th></tr>
<tr><td>12 lb</td><td colspan="4" rowspan="3">Methylphenidate is not recommended for very young children. Most children are not medicated until kindergarten.</td></tr>
<tr><td>22 lb</td></tr>
<tr><td>33 lb</td></tr>
<tr><td>44 lb</td><td>1\½</td><td></td><td colspan="2" rowspan="3">These forms are used once final dosage is reached. The sustained release form lasts 4-6 hours and is not always as effective as 2 doses.</td></tr>
<tr><td>66 lb</td><td>2\1</td><td>1\½</td></tr>
<tr><td>88 lb</td><td>2 or 3\1</td><td>1\½</td></tr>
</table>

SIDE EFFECTS

The most common side effect of treatment with methylphenidate (Ritalin) is loss of appetite, followed by a voracious appetite when the medication wears off. While few children on methylphenidate are obese and many become slimmer, weight loss is unusual and growth effects due to loss of appetite are minimal. When used for children who truly benefit from the drug, the improvement in social and academic function far outweighs the growth effects.

Occasional adverse reactions include dizziness, headache, rash, heart palpitations, changes in pulse rate and blood pressure, and nausea. Rare cases of toxic psychosis have been reported. Tourette's syndrome may be precipitated or worsened by this or any stimulant drug. Depression or mood disorders can also occur in some children. If your child experiences any of these effects, discontinue use at once and consult your pediatrician.

IMPORTANT PRECAUTIONS

It cannot be overemphasized that the dose for stimulants such as methylphenidate (Ritalin) needs to be individualized. These drugs have a threshold effect. That means that the drug may have no significant effects until the threshold level is reached. At that level the drug is fully effective, and increasing the dose only runs the risk of causing side effects without any significant therapeutic benefit.

Children who are treated with methylphenidate should be monitored by individuals skilled in the management of the disorder. Methylphenidate is only used to treat attention deficit disorders, with or without hyperactivity. It is not useful for other types of learning or behavior disorders. Proper diagnosis before treatment is begun is therefore extremely important.

Methylphenidate is not recommended for the treatment of children who exhibit extreme anxiety, tension, or agitation, as it may aggravate these conditions.

Children who require long-term therapy with methylphenidate should be monitored for potential growth problems.

Methylphenidate may increase the concentration of anticonvulsants such as phenobarbital and phenytoin and some antidepressants, so dosages should be adjusted accordingly. Be certain to tell your child's pediatrician about all medications that you are giving your child, in order to properly balance drug interactions.

METHYLPREDNISOLONE

BRAND NAMES

Duralone, Medrol

GENERAL INFORMATION

Methylprednisolone is an oral corticosteroid prescribed to reduce inflammation and relieve symptoms in a variety of childhood disorders, including severe asthma and allergic reactions. Since oral corticosteroids have potentially serious side effects, however, they are only used when other alternatives—notably oral antihistamines and topical corticosteroids—prove ineffective.

Methylprednisolone is prescribed with extreme caution. Utilization of methylprednisolone for five- to seven-day periods (or bursts) is very helpful in reducing inflammation. When used for short periods, methylprednisolone causes very few problems. There is occasional bloating and increased appetite with doses of five to seven days.

Long-term use of methylprednisolone can increase a child's risk of very serious health problems, including stunted growth, obesity, osteoporosis, a weakened immune system, and acne. Use of methylprednisolone or any other oral steroid for more than a week or on a chronic basis requires close medical supervision by a physician skilled in steroid use.

DOSAGE AND ADMINISTRATION

Methylprednisolone is available for children in tablet form. The dose can be given as a single daily dose or divided up into four doses, at the prescriber's discretion.

Doses given are the therapeutic range for the suppression of acute inflammatory situations. Daily use of this medication for more than one week is specific to the condition and is not covered here. The dose range here is wide but the higher dosages are most often used. Your physician may adjust the dosage for children who fall in-between the following weights. The dose given here is for twice daily dosage. The medication can be given in as few as one dose or as many as four doses daily. The total daily dose is unchanged.

	2 mg tablets	4 mg tablets	8 mg tablets	16 mg tablets
12 lb	—	—	—	—
22 lb	—	—	—	—
33 lb	2–6	1–3	1	—
44 lb	3–7	2–3	1	—
66 lb	4–10	2–5	1–2	1
88 lb	5–15	3–7	2–4	1–2

SIDE EFFECTS

The most common side effects of treatment with methylprednisolone are increased appetite, bloating, and weight gain. The effects can be counteracted to some extent by reducing sodium in your child's diet (for instance, avoid sodium-packed cured meats and processed foods) and increasing potassium intake (bananas are an excellent source of potassium).

The incidence of side effects due to treatment with methylprednisolone increases with dosage, frequency, and length of therapy.

Stunted growth in children can be the most serious adverse reaction to long-term treatment with methylprednisolone, and can lead to bone loss. Treatment on alternate days may minimize this dangerous side effect.

Long-term use of methylprednisolone may also compromise a child's immune system, increasing susceptibility to fungal, bacterial, and viral infections.

Bone fractures, high blood pressure, flushing, dizziness, mood changes, insomnia, headache, stomach upset, muscle weakness, and rounding of the face have all been associated with long-term treatment with methylprednisolone. Your child's pediatrician or consulting specialist should monitor your child for the complications of long-term therapy that requires the use of steroids.

IMPORTANT PRECAUTIONS

Treatment with methylprednisolone may trigger many side effects, and therefore requires very close supervision by your child's pediatrician. You should always administer methylprednisolone to your child exactly as prescribed by your pediatrician, who will recommend the lowest possible effective dosage. Parents should not start therapy with methylprednisolone unless directed specifically by their pediatrician.

If your child has diabetes, tuberculosis, or a pre-existing psychiatric illness, methylprednisolone can aggravate these conditions and may not be an appropriate medication.

Because treatment with methylprednisolone can make a child more susceptible to infection, a child should be vaccinated during treatment with methylprednisolone only under careful medical supervision, and only if necessary.

METHYLPREDNISONE ACETATE

See Corticosteroids, Topical

METRONIDAZOLE

BRAND NAME

Flagyl

GENERAL INFORMATION

Metronidazole, more commonly known as Flagyl, is prescribed to treat susceptible protozoan (a form of parasite) and bacterial infections in children. It is an effective remedy for problems such as amebiasis, vaginitis, giardiasis, and anaerobic bacterial infections. Metronidazole works by killing the organisms responsible for the infection.

In the past, pediatricians have been reluctant to use metronidazole in children because it has been associated with bladder cancer in laboratory rats. Currently, most experts feel the drug can be used safely in children.

DOSAGE AND ADMINISTRATION

Metronidazole is available for children in suspension and tablet form. Medication is usually administered three times a day for seven to ten days. Dosages here are for the treatment of common infections, such as vaginitis and giardiasis. Treatment for amebiasis requires a dose three times as large. Treatment for abdominal infections and inflammatory bowel disease are not covered here. Your physician may adjust the dosage for children who fall in-between the following weights. Metronidazole is given in three doses daily.

	100 mg suspension*	250 mg tablets
12 lb	¼ tsp	—
22 lb	½ tsp	—
33 lb	¾ tsp	—
44 lb	1 tsp	½
66 lb	1½ tsp	½
88 lb	—	1

*Your pharmacist must make this, according to instructions contained in the *Handbook of Extemporaneous Formulations,* published by the American Society of Hospital Pharmacists.

SIDE EFFECTS

The most common side effects of treatment with metronidazole (Flagyl) are nausea and stomach distress. Less common are vomiting and diarrhea. If one or more of these complaints become severe, discontinue use and consult your pediatrician.

Less common adverse reactions include dryness of the mouth, an unpleasant metallic taste, hives, burning upon urination, darkening of the urine, headache, dizziness, and fever. *Rare but more serious adverse effects* include central nervous system disturbances such as seizures and numbness and tingling in arms and legs. If your child experiences any of these effects, discontinue use at once and consult your pediatrician.

IMPORTANT PRECAUTIONS

Metronidazole (Flagyl) should not be taken in large doses for prolonged periods because of concerns, however remote, of its carcinogenic potential.

Many drugs—such as oral anticoagulants, cimetidine, rifampin, phenobarbital, and phenytoin—interact with metronidazole. Be certain to tell your child's pediatrician about all medications that you are giving your child, in order to properly balance drug interactions.

MINOCYCLINE

BRAND NAME

Minocin

GENERAL INFORMATION

Minocycline is a form of tetracycline prescribed to treat susceptible bacterial infections in children. These include ameobic dysentery, cholera, respiratory infections, acne, certain sexually transmitted diseases, and some urinary tract infections. Minocycline is generally not recommended for children under the age of eight, since it may cause yellow staining of developing permanent teeth.

DOSAGE AND ADMINISTRATION

Minocycline should not be taken with milk or dairy products, but may be taken with nondairy meals. It is available for children in suspension, tablet, and capsule form.

	50 mg oral suspension	50 mg tablets and capsules	100 mg tablets and capsules
12 lb.	Not recommended	Not recommended	Not recommended
22 lb	Not recommended	Not recommended	Not recommended
33 lb	Not recommended	Not recommended	Not recommended
44 lb	Not recommended	Not recommended	Not recommended
66 lb	1¼ tsp	1	—
88 lb	2 tsp	2	1

SIDE EFFECTS

The most common side effects of treatment with minocycline are nausea and vomiting. Sensitivity reactions, such as rashes and fever, also occur. If one or more of these complaints become severe, discontinue use and consult your pediatrician.

Less frequent adverse reactions are photosensitivity and consequent rashes from sun exposure. Dizziness and vertigo have been reported. If your child experiences any of these effects, discontinue use at once and consult your pediatrician.

IMPORTANT PRECAUTIONS

Minocycline is not an appropriate remedy for children under eight, since it may cause permanent discoloration of adult teeth while they are being formed.

Many drugs—such as penicillin, iron-containing preparations, and antacids—interact with minocycline. Be certain to tell your child's pediatrician about all medications that you are giving your child, in order to properly balance drug interactions.

MUPIROCIN

BRAND NAME

Bactroban

GENERAL INFORMATION

Mupirocin is prescribed for the topical treatment of susceptible bacterial skin infections in children. It is commonly recommended for impetigo. Mupirocin is the only antibacterial ointment that is truly effective against common skin infections.

DOSAGE AND ADMINISTRATION

Mupirocin is for external use only. Apply a small amount to the affected area up to three times daily.

SIDE EFFECTS

Side effects to treatment with mupirocin are uncommon.

Infrequent serious side effects or *adverse reactions* include itching, burning, stinging, redness, and inflammation. If your child experiences any of these effects, discontinue use at once and consult your pediatrician.

IMPORTANT PRECAUTIONS

If mupirocin does not clear up a skin infection in three to five days, or if the infection worsens, notify your pediatrician. Prolonged use of mupirocin may select out bacteria that are resistant to it.

NITROFURANTOIN

BRAND NAMES

Macrobid, Macrodantin

GENERAL INFORMATION

Nitrofurantoin is an antibacterial medication prescribed to treat urinary tract infections in children. Since treatment with nitrofurantoin can lead to a number of side effects (some of them serious), your pediatrician should closely monitor your child's condition during administration of this drug.

DOSAGE AND ADMINISTRATION

Nitrofurantoin should not be given to children under one month of age. It is best administered with meals to improve absorption.

Nitrofurantoin is available for children in suspension, capsule, and tablet form. Dosage is based on a dose of 0.7 mg per pound. This is an average dose. Doses of one-third more or less are within the appropriate range. Your physician may adjust the dosage for children who fall in-between the following weights.

	25 mg suspension	25 mg capsules	50 mg capsules & tablets	100 mg capsules & tablets
12 lb	⅓ tsp	—	—	—
22 lb	⅔ tsp	—	—	—
33 lb	1 tsp	1	—	—
44 lb	1¼ tsp	—	—	—
66 lb	2 tsp	2	—	—
88 lb	—	2–4	1–2	1

SIDE EFFECTS

Common side effects from treatment with nitrofurantoin include anorexia, nausea, and vomiting. If one or more of these complaints become severe, discontinue use and consult your pediatrician.

Less common side effects are diarrhea, fever, rashes, chills, headache, dizziness, drowsiness, and vertigo. Children with a history of asthma may experience asthma attacks, and lung problems in general are a possible complication of treatment with nitrofurantoin. In rare cases, jaundice may develop. If your child experiences any of these effects, discontinue use at once and consult your pediatrician.

IMPORTANT PRECAUTIONS

Nitrofurantoin should be used with caution in children who have severe kidney problems, anemia, or diabetes.

Medications such as antacids interact with nitrofurantoin. Be certain to tell your child's pediatrician about all medications that you are giving your child, in order to properly balance drug interactions.

NYSTATIN

BRAND NAMES

Nilstat, Mycostatin

GENERAL INFORMATION

Nystatin is an antibiotic prescribed for the treatment of fungus infections in children. Fungal infections may infect the mouth, as in thrush (which is characterized by milky-white patches), the skin, mucous membranes, intestines, or genital area. A fungal diaper rash may appear red, raw, and pimply.

Nystatin works by preventing the growth and reproduction of fungus.

DOSAGE AND ADMINISTRATION

Nystatin is available orally in suspension form, and topically as cream or powder. The topical forms are also available in combination with cortisone creams.

Nystatin is not absorbed into the body and dosage is therefore not related significantly to weight. A smaller dose is given to newborns in consideration of their size.

	Suspension	Topical cream or powder
12 lb	1.0 ml 4 times daily	Apply to affected area 2–4 times daily
22 lb	1–2 ml 4 times daily	Apply to affected area 2–4 times daily
33 lb	1–2 ml 4 times daily	Apply to affected area 2–4 times daily
44 lb	1–2 ml 4 times daily	Apply to affected area 2–4 times daily
66 lb	1–2 ml 4 times daily	Apply to affected area 2–4 times daily
88 lb	1–2 ml 4 times daily	Apply to affected area 2–4 times daily

SIDE EFFECTS

Side effects of treatment with nystatin are uncommon. In rare cases, nausea, vomiting, and diarrhea may develop after treatment with oral medication. Local irritation has also been observed, rarely, after topical administration. If your child experiences any of these effects, discontinue use at once and consult your pediatrician.

IMPORTANT PRECAUTIONS

For treatment with nystatin to be effective, it is important to follow the entire course of medication prescribed by your pediatrician. Nystatin should not be given to children who have experienced a sensitivity or allergic reaction to it in the past.

PEMOLINE

BRAND NAME

Cylert

GENERAL INFORMATION

Pemoline is prescribed to treat the behavioral syndrome known as attention deficit hyperactivity disorder (ADHD) in children. Although pemoline is a mild central nervous system stimulant, it acts to calm the hyperactive child, contributing to the management of overactivity and lengthening the attention spans of hyperactive children. Drugs that are used to manage attention deficit disorders should be integrated within a complete program of psychological, social, and educational treatment. Pemoline is not an appropriate medication for children under the age of six.

DOSAGE AND ADMINISTRATION

	18.75 mg tablets	37.5 mg tablets/ chewable tablets	75 mg tablets
12 lb	Pemoline is not recommended for children less than 6 years of age.		
22 lb			
33 lb			
44 lb			
66 lb	Begin with a dose of 37.5 mg daily in the morning and increase by 18.75 mg until desired effect is obtained. Usual dosages are 56.25–75 mg daily. Maximum dosage is 112.5 mg. Weight is not a significant factor in dosage.		
88 lb			

Pemoline is available for children in tablet form. Unlike other drugs used to treat attention deficit disorders, this medication is given in a single morning dose. A second dose is never given.

SIDE EFFECTS

The most common side effects of treatment with pemoline are insomnia and anorexia. Insomnia may pass without intervention, or may be reversed through an adjustment of dosage.

Anorexia and weight loss may result during early therapy with pemoline—although weight gain subsequently occurs and total weight evens out after three to six months of therapy.

Less frequent adverse reactions include dizziness, drowsiness, headache, depression, hallucinations, rash, and nausea. If your child experiences any of these effects, discontinue use at once and consult your pediatrician.

IMPORTANT PRECAUTIONS

A rare delayed reaction to pemoline is liver failure, which can be fatal. The liver function of children should therefore be monitored closely during treatment.

Long-term use of pemoline has also been associated with rare instances of growth retardation. This effect, however, appears temporary.

PENICILLIN V POTASSIUM

BRAND NAMES

Pen-Vee K, V-Cillin K

GENERAL INFORMATION

Penicillin is an antibiotic commonly prescribed to treat a wide range of bacterial infections in children, including infections of the upper and lower respiratory tract, dental infections, rheumatic fever, and scarlet fever. Penicillin works by weakening susceptible bacterial cell walls, resulting in the death of infectious organisms. Because humans possess a different kind of cell wall, it has no effect on normal human cell walls. A special type of penicillin known as benzathine penicillin is a long-acting form of the drug, which can be used to give low levels of penicillin for long periods of time (twenty-one days).

Penicillin is only effective against susceptible *bacterial*—not viral, parasitic, or fungal—infections. Your child will usually show signs of improvement following two or three days of treatment, and should be well on the road to recovery in four to five days. If toxic symptoms or discomfort continue after this time, consult your pediatrician. Your child may be suffering from an infection that is resistant to penicillin, and the doctor may want to see your child and/or prescribe an alternate treatment.

DOSAGE AND ADMINISTRATION

Penicillin should be given one hour before or two hours after meals for maximum absorption.

Penicillin is available for children as an oral solution or in tablets. It is administered four times a day, as close to every six hours as is practical. (Benzathine penicillin, on the other hand, is given as a single dose.)

The dosage of penicillin given is based on a dose of 23 mg per pound. This is the upper range of the recommended dose, and is appropriate with emerging resistance to penicillin among bacteria that had formerly been very sensitive to it. Your physician may adjust the dosage for children who fall in-between the following weights.

	125 mg oral solution	250 mg oral solution	250 mg tablets	500 mg tablets
12 lb	½ tsp	—	—	—
22 lb	1 tsp	½ tsp	—	—
33 lb	1½ tsp	¾ tsp	—	—
44 lb	—	1 tsp	1	—
66 lb	—	1½ tsp	2*	1*
88 lb	—	2	2	1

*This dose is higher than is usually recommended. There is no overdose possibility with penicillin, so erring on the side of excess is acceptable.

SIDE EFFECTS

The most common side effects of treatment with penicillin are allergic skin rashes. If a skin rash becomes severe, discontinue use and consult your pediatrician.

Less frequent adverse reactions include hives, swelling of the body, joint pain, and swollen lymph nodes. If your child experiences any of these effects, discontinue use at once and consult your pediatrician.

In rare cases of respiratory difficulty or shock, take your child to the emergency room immediately.

IMPORTANT PRECAUTIONS

For treatment with penicillin to be effective—and to prevent infection from recurring—it's important to follow the entire course of medication prescribed by your pediatrician, even after your child's symptoms have diminished or disappeared. This is especially important with treatment of strep throat.

Penicillin should be used with caution in children who have a history of severe allergic reactions to many substances. A minor dot-like rash, especially one that occurs two to four days after treatment with penicillin has begun, is more likely to be viral than allergic. Hives that appear after each dose, on the other hand, are probably allergic reactions. If the reaction is mild, your health care provider may try penicillin again at a later date. If your child has had a severe reaction to penicillin, cephalosporins should be given with close medical supervision.

Skin tests are available for penicillin allergy. Most experts, however, restrict their use of skin tests to individuals who have had a worrisome reaction in the past that may or may not have been due to penicillin.

Other drugs interact with penicillin. Be certain to tell your child's pediatrician about all medications that you are giving your child, in order to properly balance drug interactions.

PHENOBARBITAL

BRAND NAMES

Barbita, Luminal, PBR/12, Sedadrops, Solfoton

GENERAL INFORMATION

Phenobarbital is one of the most useful and widely prescribed anticonvulsant drugs to treat and prevent seizure disorders in children. Yet, much has changed in the use of seizure medications in the last few years.

Following a seizure in your child, the pediatrician may conduct tests to determine the underlying cause. Phenobarbital is, in many cases, the initial drug prescribed to treat epileptic seizures or convulsions in very young children.

In the recent past, phenobarbital was also very commonly prescribed for febrile (nonepileptic) seizures in children. Febrile seizures can occur in children between three months and five years of age, and are usually due to a rapid rise or fall in body temperature, rather than simply a high fever. Contrary to popular opinion, febrile seizures, while alarming to parents, do not cause brain damage in children. As a result, most children with febrile seizures are no longer medicated.

Because phenobarbital interferes with learning and can cause behavior problems, its use is now limited to infants. Other drugs, such as valproic acid and carbamezepine, are more commonly used for children with recurrent seizures. Chronic use of seizure medication (for more than two years) is reserved for special situations. If your child has been prescribed seizure medications such as phenobarbital for more than 2 years without EEG (brain wave) testing, consult a pediatric neurologist to determine if these drugs are needed.

DOSAGE AND ADMINISTRATION

Phenobarbital is available for children in elixir or tablet form. The dose of phenobarbital is determined primarily by the level in the bloodstream; doses given here are usual

	15 mg elixir	20 mg elixir	15 mg tablets	30 mg tablets
12 lb	1 tsp twice daily*	⅔ tsp twice daily*	—	—
22 lb	2 tsp twice daily*	1½ tsp twice daily*	—	—
33 lb	3 tsp twice daily*	2¼ tsp twice daily*	3*	—
44 lb	4 tsp twice daily*	3 tsp twice daily*	4*	2*
66 lb	4 tsp twice daily*	3 tsp twice daily*	4*	2*
88 lb	—	—	2–4**	1–2**

*Can be given as a double dose once daily, at bedtime.

**The dose by weight for phenobarbital can decrease with age and puberty. There are exceptions. Keep in mind the dose of phenobarbital is determined by blood drug levels; weight is only one factor.

doses. Differences in how the drug is metabolized may result in a significant variation of the effective dose from one child to another.

SIDE EFFECTS

Common side effects from treatment with phenobarbital include hyperactivity, irritability, excitement, and sleep disturbances. These may occur in approximately 25 percent of the children who are given this drug. Treatment in these cases should be discontinued, and phenobarbital should be replaced with an alternative anticonvulsant.

Less frequent adverse reactions to treatment with phenobarbital are skin rashes and anemia. As with common complaints, discontinue treatment at once and consult your pediatrician.

IMPORTANT PRECAUTIONS

Since phenobarbital can cause significant side effects in children, careful monitoring of blood levels by your pediatrician is essential.

The discontinuation of treatment with phenobarbital should be accomplished on a gradual basis, according to the exact instructions of your pediatrician, so as not to aggravate seizures.

Many drugs interact with phenobarbital. These drugs include griseofulvin, theophylline, antidepressants, valproic acid (Depakote), and methylphenidate (Ritalin). Phenobarbital is sometimes prescribed in combination with another anticonvulsant (such as phenytoin (Dilantin) or valproic acid (Depakote)) to increase its effectiveness. Phenobarbital may reduce the effectiveness of griseofulvin and certain antibiotics such as tetracycline. It may increase the effects of corticosteroids.

Be certain to tell your child's pediatrician about all medications that you are giving your child, in order to properly balance drug interactions.

PHENYTOIN

BRAND NAME

Dilantin

GENERAL INFORMATION

Phenytoin is an anticonvulsant drug prescribed to treat and prevent seizure disorders in children. Although phenytoin is an effective therapy, it has a number of potential adverse side effects. Any drug that prevents seizures has the potential to interfere with learning and with behavior. This effect has been well-documented with phenytoin and phenobarbital, and to a lesser extent with other drugs such as carbamazepine and valproic acid.

DOSAGE AND ADMINISTRATION

Phenytoin is available for children as suspensions, tablets, and sustained release preparations. Dosage of phenytoin varies with age, with older children requiring less by weight than younger children. The doses given here are for seizure control. (Doses for heart rhythm disorders are approxi-

	50 mg chewable tablets	125 mg suspension	100 mg capsules	100 mg sustained-release*
12 lb	—	.85–1.1 cc	—	—
22 lb	—	1.6–2.0 cc	—	—
33 lb	1–1½	½–⅔ tsp	—	—
44 lb	1½–2	⅔–¾ tsp	—	1–2, once daily*
66 lb	2	¾–1 tsp	1	2, once daily*
88 lb	2½–3	1–1¼	1	2–3, once daily*

*This is the only formulation that can be given once daily (at bedtime). All others are given twice daily.

mately the same.) Where appropriate, a dosage range is given.

Phenytoin is given twice daily, with the exception of the sustained-release formulations, which can be given once a day at bedtime.

SIDE EFFECTS

The most common side effect from treatment with phenytoin (Dilantin) is skin rash, although it is rarely serious. If a skin rash becomes severe, discontinue use and consult your pediatrician.

Overgrowth of the gums is another common problem in children who are treated with phenytoin; this condition, where the gums grow to cover the teeth, is both cosmetically unacceptable and also creates a situation where gums can easily become infected. Even good oral hygiene will only eliminate secondary infections—it cannot prevent the initial condition. If this problem becomes severe, speak to your pediatrician about the possibility of replacing phenytoin with an alternative anticonvulsant.

A less common side effect of treatment with phenytoin is hirsutism (excess hair growth). If this problem becomes severe, consult your pediatrician.

Rare but very serious reactions include Stevens-Johnson syndrome (a severe hive-like eruption of the skin associated with inflammation of the membranes of the eyes and mouth), bleeding problems, unsteady gait, jerky eye movements, hepatitis (often indicated by severe fatigue and abdominal pain), lupus (usually accompanied by a butterfly-shaped rash on the face), and bone marrow and lymph problems. If you suspect that your child is experiencing any of these effects, discontinue use at once and consult your pediatrician.

IMPORTANT PRECAUTIONS

Since phenytoin (Dilantin) can cause significant side effects in children, careful monitoring of blood levels by your pediatrician is essential.

The discontinuation of treatment with phenytoin should be accomplished on a gradual basis, according to the exact instruction of your pediatrician, so as not to aggravate seizures.

Many drugs interact with phenytoin. Phenytoin is often prescribed in combination with the anticonvulsant phenobarbital in order to increase its effectiveness. Yet phenytoin, when taken with the anticonvulsant carbamazepine, decreases the effectiveness of both drugs.

There is little evidence that two anticonvulsants are better than one for severe epilepsy. When two anticonvulsants, such as phenytoin and valproic acid, are prescribed together, the effect is complex; the level of phenytoin in the body can be either increased or decreased through interaction with valproic acid. This is one of the reasons why all combinations of anticonvulsants are now used only in the most extreme of circumstances.

The concentration of phenytoin in the body may be increased—with a resulting increase in side effects—when it is taken in conjunction with other drugs such as cimetidine (Tagamet), isoniazid, and trimethoprim.

Phenytoin may also reduce the effectiveness of oral anticoagulants and certain antibiotics, such as tetracycline.

Be certain to tell your child's pediatrician about all medications that you are giving your child, in order to properly balance drug interactions.

POLYMYXIN B, NEOMYCIN SULFATE, AND GRAMICIDIN (EYE MEDICATION)

BRAND NAME

Neosporin

GENERAL INFORMATION

Neosporin is a combination of three antibiotics that is prescribed in eyedrop or ointment form to treat eye infections in children. Eye problems such as conjunctivitis, or pinkeye, are irritating to children and extremely contagious, but prompt treatment will ordinarily clear them up within a day or two.

DOSAGE AND ADMINISTRATION

Neosporin is available for children as eyedrops or ointment. Apply two to three drops or ½-inch ribbon of ointment to the affected eye two to four times a day as directed. Ointments are generally easier to apply in young children. Pull down the lower lid and apply the ribbon to the inside of the lower lid.

SIDE EFFECTS

Side effects are uncommon, since Neosporin administered in this manner is not a systemic drug. Occasionally a rash may develop around the eye if drops fall on the skin. If the rash becomes severe, discontinue use and consult your pediatrician.

IMPORTANT PRECAUTIONS

Neomycin is a highly allergenic drug. If the conjunctivitis persists or worsens, an allergy to neomycin may be the cause.

POLYMYXIN B, NEOMYCIN SULFATE, AND HYDROCORTISONE (EARDROPS)

BRAND NAME

Cortisporin Otic Solution

GENERAL INFORMATION

Cortisporin Otic Solution is prescribed to treat external bacterial ear infections in children (otis externa or swimmer's ear). In Cortisporin, two broad-spectrum antibiotics are joined with a corticosteroid, so that the bacterial infection will be cured while symptomatic inflammation and itching are relieved.

DOSAGE AND ADMINISTRATION

Before administering eardrops, warm the bottle of solution slightly by holding under a stream of hot water; then test a few drops on your hand to make sure they are not too hot.

Next, lie your child sideways across your lap, and administer the correct number of drops into the ear (three drops three or four times daily). Aim at the wall of the ear canal. Keep your child still for a minute or two, so eardrops do not drain out. Never share eardroppers or ear medication, and be sure not to touch the tip of the eardropper, which may be contaminated.

SIDE EFFECTS

The most common side effect from the antibiotic neomycin in Cortisporin Otic Solution is local irritation, mimicking the original problem. If irritation or sensitivity to neomycin develops, treatment should be discontinued.

Other adverse reactions are uncommon, but include irritation or sensitivity to any of the ingredients in Cortisporin.

If your child experiences any adverse effects, discontinue use and consult your pediatrician.

IMPORTANT PRECAUTIONS

Any preparation containing a corticosteroid such as hydrocortisone should not be given to children who have herpes simplex or chicken pox. In general, Cortisporin is an antibiotic that is an effective treatment for external ear infections caused by bacteria; it is not an appropriate medication for viral or fungal external ear infections.

For treatment with Cortisporin to be effective—and to prevent infection from recurring—it's important to follow the entire course of medication prescribed by your pediatrician, even after your child's symptoms have diminished or disappeared.

PREDNISONE/ PREDNISOLONE

BRAND NAMES

Deltasone, Meticorten, Orasone, Pediapred, Prelome

GENERAL INFORMATION

Prednisone is an oral corticosteroid commonly prescribed to treat a wide variety of inflammatory and allergic conditions. It is an especially effective medication for severe asthma, as well as for blood disorders, lung diseases, and skin problems. Prednisone is often prescribed on a short-term basis to reverse allergic reactions to foods, medications, or poison ivy.

While prednisone is very effective, it can lead to major side effects and is prescribed with extreme caution. Utilization of prednisone for five- to seven-day periods (or bursts) is very helpful in reducing inflammation. When used for these short periods, prednisone causes very few problems, although there may be occasional bloating and increased appetite with doses of five to seven days.

Long-term use of prednisone can increase a child's risk of very serious health problems, including stunted growth, obesity, acne, and a weakened immune system. Use of prednisone or any other oral steroid for more than a week or on a chronic basis requires close medical supervision by a physician skilled in steroid use.

DOSAGE AND ADMINISTRATION

Prednisone and prednisolone are equivalent drugs and are discussed together here. When the medication is given for less than a week, the dose may remain the same or start high and gradually be "tapered" downward in stairstep fashion. Either approach is appropriate.

When used for longer than a week, your pediatrician will gradually adjust dosage to the lowest possible effective level for your child. Prednisone may also be prescribed on alternate days in order to minimize side effects and retain your child's natural ability to produce its hormonal equivalent. If prednisone is prescribed for more than one week, dosage should be gradually withdrawn.

Prednisone is available in suspension or tablet form. The dose may be as little as once daily or as often as four times

	5 mg suspension (Pediapred)	15 mg suspension (Prelome)	5 mg tablets	10 mg tablets	20 mg tablets
12 lb	½–1 tsp	—	—	—	—
22 lb	1–2 tsp	⅓–⅔ tsp	—	—	—
33 lb	1½–3 tsp	½–1 tsp	—	—	—
44 lb	2–4 tsp	⅔ tsp–1⅓ tsp	2–4	1–2	—
66 lb	3–6 tsp	1–2 tsp	3–6	2–3	1–2
88 lb	—	—	4–8	2–4	1–2

Note: Some providers will decrease the dose in the last few days. If the dose is given for less than a week, this is unnecessary, but still a common and perfectly acceptable practice.

daily without any difference in effect. Most practitioners dose twice daily. Doses given here are also twice daily. (You may calculate other regimens with simple mathematics.)

Dosage here is based on a range of 0.45 to 9 mg per pound as a total daily dose, and relate to short-term suppression of immunological/inflammatory problems such as asthma. The medication is usually given for three to seven days. Dosage for more than a week requires close medical supervision and reduced doses, and is not covered in this chart. Your physician may adjust the dosage for children who fall in-between the weights in the chart on page 179.

SIDE EFFECTS

The most common side effects of extended treatment with prednisone are increased appetite, bloating, and weight gain. The effects can be counteracted to some extent by reducing sodium in your child's diet (for instance, avoid sodium-packed cured meats and processed foods) and increasing potassium intake (bananas are an excellent source of potassium).

The incidence of side effects due to treatment with prednisone increases with dosage, frequency, and length of therapy.

Stunted growth in children can be the most serious adverse reaction to long-term treatment with prednisone, and can lead to bone loss. Treatment on alternate days may minimize this dangerous side effect.

Long-term use of prednisone may also compromise a child's immune system, making him or her more susceptible to fungal, bacterial, and viral infections.

Bone fractures, high blood pressure, flushing, dizziness, mood changes, insomnia, headache, stomach upset, muscle weakness, and rounding of the face have all been associated with extended treatment with prednisone. If your child experiences any of these effects, discontinue use at once and consult your pediatrician.

IMPORTANT PRECAUTIONS

Treatment with prednisone may trigger many side effects and therefore requires very close supervision by your child's pediatrician. You should always administer prednisone to your child exactly as prescribed by your pediatrician, who will recommend the lowest possible effective dosage.

If your child has diabetes, tuberculosis, or a pre-existing psychiatric illness, prednisone may not be an appropriate medication. Prednisone can aggravate these conditions.

Because treatment with prednisone can make a child more susceptible to infection, a child should be vaccinated during treatment with prednisone only under careful medical supervision, and only if necessary.

Most physicians use prednisone and methylprednisolone interchangeably. The differences are that methylprednisolone is 25 percent more powerful than the same dose of prednisone, and is more expensive.

PROCHLORPERAZINE

BRAND NAME

Compazine

GENERAL INFORMATION

Prochlorperazine is an antiemetic medication; antiemetic medications are prescribed to treat nausea and vomiting. Caution should be exercised in the administration of prochlorperazine to children. Many pediatricians today feel that the management of vomiting as part of childhood illness should not involve the use of drugs. An exception to this is vomiting that occurs after cancer chemotherapy.

DOSAGE AND ADMINISTRATION

Prochlorperazine is available for children as rectal suppositories. Prochlorperazine is not an appropriate medication for children under age two.

Prochlorperazine should be administered every six to eight hours *only as needed.* Your physician may adjust the dosage for children who fall in-between the following weights.

	2.5 mg suppository	5 mg suppository
12 lb	Contraindicated	Contraindicated
22 lb	½*	—
33 lb	½*	—
44 lb	1	—
66 lb	1	—
88 lb	—	1

*Suppositories must be cut lengthwise, because medication may settle unevenly in the suppository during manufacture.

SIDE EFFECTS

The most common side effects of treatment with prochlorperazine are nervousness and excitability. Drowsiness, dizziness, and skin problems occasionally occur. Side effects are usually associated with large doses of prochlorperazine, but they may also appear suddenly as a result of even moderate doses, especially in children. If one or more of these complaints become severe, discontinue use and consult your pediatrician.

More serious but rarely occurring side effects include low blood pressure, twitches, and rather dramatic involuntary muscle spasms that contort the body may occur. If your child experiences any of these effects, discontinue use at once and consult your pediatrician.

IMPORTANT PRECAUTIONS

Prochlorperazine should not be given to children under the age of two. It should not be prescribed for children who are undergoing surgery or children who are suspected of having Reye syndrome.

Other drugs—such as the anticonvulsants carbamazepine (Tegretol) and phenytoin (Dilantin)—may interact with prochlorperazine. Be certain to tell your child's pediatrician about all medications that you are giving your child, in order to properly balance drug interactions.

PROMETHAZINE

BRAND NAME

Phenergan

GENERAL INFORMATION

Promethazine is prescribed as an antihistamine, as an antiemitic agent, and for motion sickness in children. As an antihistamine, promethazine is used to treat hay fever, hives, rashes, and itching in children. It may also control motion sickness, nausea, and vomiting, and can be helpful in cases of penicillin sensitivity and allergic reactions to certain foods.

Antihistamines work by blocking the action of histamine released from specialized allergy cells called mast cells. Histamine is the substance that most commonly causes itching and inflammation, and reactions to histamine can lead to difficulty in breathing due to narrowing and inflammation of the airways and increased mucous secretion.

DOSAGE AND ADMINISTRATION

Promethazine is available for children in syrup, tablet, and suppository form. Suppositories are not appropriate for children under two, and the use of tablets is reserved for children who weigh at least 66 pounds.

As an antihistamine, promethazine should be administered three times a day. For vomiting, the medication is given every four to six hours as needed. For motion sickness, the drug is given every twelve hours, starting ½–1 hour before beginning travel. Your physician may adjust the dosage for children who fall in-between these weights.

DOSAGES FOR ANTIHISTAMINE USE

	6.25 mg syrup	25 mg syrup	12.5 mg suppository	25 mg suppository	12.5 mg tablets	25 mg tablets
12 lb	—	—	—	—	—	—
22 lb	1 cc	—	—	—	—	—
33 lb	¼ tsp	—	—	—	—	—
44 lb	⅓ tsp	—	—	—	—	—
66 lb	½ tsp	—	—	—	—	—
88 lb	⅔ tsp	—	—	—	½	—

DOSAGE FOR VOMITING, NAUSEA AND TRAVEL SICKNESS

	6.25 mg syrup	12.5 mg suppository	25 mg suppository	12.5 mg tablets	25 mg tablets
12 lb	—	—	—	—	—
22 lb	½–¾ tsp	—	—	—	—
33 lb	½–1¼ tsp	½	—	—	—
44 lb	¾–1½ tsp	½	—	—	—
66 lb	1¼–2½ tsp	1	—	1	—
88 lb	1⅔–3 tsp	1	1	1–2	1

SIDE EFFECTS

The most common side effect of treatment with promethazine is drowsiness.

Occasionally *adverse reactions* such as photosensitivity—unusual sensitivity to sunlight—may develop. If your child experiences this effect, discontinue use and consult your pediatrician.

IMPORTANT PRECAUTIONS

Like other antihistamines, promethazine may cause drowsiness and impaired coordination. Parents might therefore choose to limit children's participation in activities such as climbing or gymnastics while taking this medication.

Other drugs may interact with promethazine. Be certain to tell your child's pediatrician about all medications that you are giving your child, in order to properly balance drug interactions.

RANITIDINE

BRAND NAME

Zantac

GENERAL INFORMATION

Ranitidine is prescribed for the short-term treatment of gastric and duodenal ulcers in children and the treatment of acid reflux in infants, as well as for hyperacidity. Like cimetidine, this drug is a histamine receptor antagonist that works by inhibiting gastric secretions. In fact, ranitidine is five to eight times more effective than cimetidine in suppressing gastric acid secretion.

DOSAGE AND ADMINISTRATION

Ranitidine is available for children in suspension or tablet form. It is administered every twelve hours, and should be taken with food and at bedtime for maximum effect.

Recommended dosages of ranitidine will depend on the nature of your child's condition. The dosage given here is 0.9 to 1.8 mg per pound. Any dose in the range is appropriate. Your physician may adjust the dosage for children who fall in-between the following weights.

	15 mg suspension	150 mg tablets
12 lb	⅓–⅔ tsp	—
22 lb	⅔–1⅓ tsp	—
33 lb	1–2 tsp	—
44 lb	1⅓–2⅔ tsp	—
66 lb	2–4 tsp	—
88 lb	2⅔–5⅓ tsp	1*

*This is an adult dose and is acceptable at this weight.

SIDE EFFECTS

Minor side effects rarely occur.

Serious adverse reactions to ranitidine include headache (sometimes severe), dizziness, sleep problems, cardiac arrhythmias, hepatitis, and blood count changes. Allergic reactions such as hives can occur. These reactions have been serious and life-threatening in a few instances. If your child experiences any of these effects, discontinue use at once and consult your pediatrician.

IMPORTANT PRECAUTIONS

None.

SULFACETAMIDE (EYE MEDICATION)

BRAND NAME

Sulamyd

GENERAL INFORMATION

Sulfacetamide is an antibacterial sulfa drug prescribed in eyedrop or ointment form to treat eye infections in children. Eye problems such as conjunctivitis, or pinkeye, are irritating to children and extremely contagious, but prompt treatment will ordinarily clear them up within a day or two.

DOSAGE AND ADMINISTRATION

Sulfacetamide is available for children as eyedrops or ointment. Apply two to three drops or ½-inch ribbon of ointment to the affected eye two to four times a day as directed. Ointments are generally easier to apply in young children. Pull down the lower lid and apply the ribbon to the inside of the lower lid.

SIDE EFFECTS

Side effects are common, since sulfacetamide is somewhat irritating. Local irritation, stinging, and burning are usual symptoms. If one or more of these complaints become severe, discontinue use and consult your pediatrician.

A severe swelling of the eyes, mucous membranes, and skin is a rare side effect of treatment with sulfacetamide. If this happens, discontinue use at once and see your pediatrician.

IMPORTANT PRECAUTIONS

Sulfacetamide should be used with caution in children who have demonstrated a previous sensitivity to sulfa drugs.

SULFISOXAZOLE (EYE MEDICATION)

BRAND NAME

Gantrisin

GENERAL INFORMATION

Sulfisoxazole is an antibacterial sulfa drug prescribed in eyedrop form to treat eye infections in children. Eye problems such as conjunctivitis, or pinkeye, are extremely contagious, but prompt treatment usually clears up infections within a day or two.

DOSAGE AND ADMINISTRATION

Sulfisoxazole is available for children as eyedrops. Apply two to three drops to the affected eye two to four times a day as directed.

SIDE EFFECTS

Frequently occurring side effects are mild burning and irritation.

There are no serious side effects.

IMPORTANT PRECAUTIONS

Sulfisoxazole should be used with caution in children who have demonstrated a previous sensitivity to sulfa drugs.

SULFISOXAZOLE (Oral)

BRAND NAME

Gantrisin

GENERAL INFORMATION

Sulfisoxazole is an antibacterial sulfa drug commonly prescribed in oral form to prevent ear infections in children.

Once a primary treatment for urinary tract infections, it has now largely been replaced by the combination of trimethoprim and sulfamethoxazole in this regard.

DOSAGE AND ADMINISTRATION

Sulfisoxazole is available for children in suspension or tablet form. The medication is given four times a day for the treatment of a urinary tract infection and two times a day for the prevention of otitis media. Your physician may adjust the dosage for children who fall in-between the following weights.

	500 mg suspension	500 mg tablets
12 lb	⅓ tsp	—
22 lb	⅔ tsp	—
33 lb	1 tsp	—
44 lb	1½ tsp	—
66 lb	2 tsp	2
88 lb	3 tsp	3

SIDE EFFECTS

Common side effects of treatment with sulfisoxazole include nausea, vomiting, diarrhea, headache, lethargy, dizziness, and depression. If one or more of these complaints become severe, discontinue use and consult your pediatrician.

Rare but very serious reactions include Stevens-Johnson syndrome (a severe hive-like eruption of the skin associated with inflammation of the membranes of the eyes and mouth), hepatitis (often indicated by severe fatigue and abdominal pain), kidney problems, hypoglycemic blood disorders, and lupus (usually accompanied by a butterfly rash on the face).

Early signs of potentially serious adverse reactions to sulfisoxazole include fever, paleness, hives, purple spots on the skin, jaundice, and joint pain. If your child experiences any of these effects, discontinue use at once and consult your pediatrician.

Life-threatening episodes of anaphylaxis (an allergic reaction characterized by sudden respiratory distress, a drop in blood pressure, and the onset of hives) have also been reported. If your child goes into anaphylaxis, call 911 and describe your child's symptoms. Do not try to take your child to the emergency room yourself unless told to do so by emergency personnel. Tell the 911 operator that you need an ambulance immediately.

IMPORTANT PRECAUTIONS

Sulfisoxazole should not be given to children under two months of age. It should not be prescribed for children who have experienced a prior sensitivity or allergy to sulfa drugs, and should be used with caution in children who have impaired liver or kidney function or a history of severe allergies.

Children who have G6PD deficiency (mostly children of African or Mediterranean ancestry) should not be given this drug, as it may cause moderately severe anemia over a very few hours.

Since sulfisoxazole may cause heightened light sensitivity, limit your child's exposure to intense sunlight or apply a broad-based sunscreen before going outside.

Many drugs—including anticonvulsants, isoniazid, penicillins, and trimethoprim—interact with sulfisoxazole. Be certain to tell your child's pediatrician about all medications that you are giving your child, in order to properly balance drug interactions.

TETRACYCLINE

BRAND NAMES

Achromycin V, Sumycin

GENERAL INFORMATION

Tetracycline is a broad-spectrum antibiotic prescribed to treat bacterial infections in children. These infections include ameobic dysentery, bronchitis, conjunctivitis, infections of the mouth, teeth, and gums, pneumonia, urinary tract infections, and acne. Tetracycline should not be given to children under 8 years old except under special circumstances because it may cause yellow staining of developing permanent teeth.

DOSAGE AND ADMINISTRATION

Tetracycline is available for children in suspension, tablet, and capsule form. It should be given four times a day. Your physician may adjust the dosage for children who fall in-between the following weights.

	125 mg suspension	250 mg tablets & capsules	500 mg tablets & capsules
12 lb	Contraindicated*	Contraindicated*	Contraindicated*
22 lb	Contraindicated*	Contraindicated*	Contraindicated*
33 lb	Contraindicated*	Contraindicated*	Contraindicated*
44 lb	Contraindicated*	Contraindicated*	Contraindicated*
66 lb	1½–3 tsp	1	—
88 lb	—	1–2	1

SIDE EFFECTS

The most common side effects of treatment with tetracycline are nausea and vomiting. If these complaints become severe, discontinue use and consult your pediatrician.

Less common serious side effects or adverse reactions to tetracycline include hives, yeast infections in the genital region, liver inflammation (usually accompanied by fatigue and jaundice), fever, photosensitivity (skin rashes from sun exposure), and chills. In rare instances, blood and kidney disorders have occurred. Signs of these include a pale complexion or spots on the skin that do not go away with pressure. If your child experiences any of these effects, discontinue use at once and consult your pediatrician.

IMPORTANT PRECAUTIONS

Tetracycline should not be given to children until their adult teeth have formed, around age eight. If given while permanent teeth are forming, it may cause permanent yellow staining of teeth.

Do not use tetracycline after the expiration date. Outdated tetracycline may be toxic to the kidneys.

Tetracycline should be used with caution in children who have a history of kidney or liver disease.

Tetracycline may cause skin rashes due to exposure to sunlight while taking this drug. Those taking tetracycline should avoid intense sunlight and use sunscreen. An alternate medication should be prescribed during periods of intense exposure.

Many drugs—such as penicillin, iron, and antacids that contain aluminum, calcium, or magnesium—interact with tetracycline. Be certain to tell your child's pediatrician about all medications that you are giving your child, in order to properly balance drug interactions.

THEOPHYLLINE

BRAND NAMES

Aerolate, Constant-T, Respbid, Slo-bid, Slo-Phyllin, Sustaine, Theo-24, Theobid, Theochron, Theo-dur, Theolair, Theovent, Uniphyl

GENERAL INFORMATION

Theophylline is a bronchodilator medication prescribed for the treatment of moderate to severe asthma in children. It works by relaxing bronchial muscles in the lungs, thus opening blocked airways and making it easier to breathe. Sustained-release theophylline preparations, such as Slo-bid and Theo-dur, are an especially effective treatment for nighttime asthma.

Recent safety concerns have focused on the large number of side effects associated with theophylline. Since the level at which theophylline is effective is very close to the level at which it has toxic effects, close monitoring of theophylline levels in the blood is necessary to prevent side effects. As safer and equally effective medications have been developed, theophylline is prescribed with greater caution than in the past.

DOSAGE AND ADMINISTRATION

The metabolism of theophylline in your child's body is affected by age, sexual maturity (metabolism slows considerably at puberty), illness, and other drugs. Close monitoring of drug levels is essential. Illness may change drug needs considerably and result in drastic alterations of blood levels and toxicity.

Theophylline is available for children in liquid and sustained-release form. The liquid is given every six hours. Sustained-release preparations are administered every twelve hours. In some children, these times must be shortened to four and eight hours, respectively. Sustained-release tablets are much preferred over liquids. Your pediatrician will carefully individualize the dosage of theophylline based on your child's needs.

	80 mg per teaspoon elixir*	80 mg per tablespoon solution*	100 mg sustained release tablets/ capsules	200 mg sustained release tablets/ capsules	300 mg sustained release tablets/ capsules
12 lb	.8 cc	½ tsp	—	—	—
22 lb	½ tsp	1½ tsp	—	—	—
33 lb	1 tsp	1 tbsp*	1	—	—
44 lb	1⅓ tsp	1⅓ tbsp*	—	1	—
66 lb	—	—	—	—	1
88 lb	—	—	—	—	1

*Please pay close attention to the difference. This is a major cause of medical problems.

SIDE EFFECTS

The most common side effects of treatment with theophylline are headache, dizziness, nervousness, nausea, vomiting, and stomach pain. Side effects are usually dose-related. If one or more of these complaints become severe, consult your pediatrician.

More serious but less frequent reactions to theophylline include fast or irregular heartbeat, persistent vomiting, and convulsions. If your child experiences any of these effects, discontinue use at once and consult your pediatrician immediately. In rare instances of overdose, convulsions and heart arrhythmias have been fatal.

IMPORTANT PRECAUTIONS

The level of theophylline in your child's blood should be closely monitored by your pediatrician. Appropriate doses of theophylline are key to ensuring that the medication is acting effectively within its therapeutic range, while at the same time reducing the incidence of side effects.

Theophylline should be prescribed with caution in children who suffer from heart problems.

A number of viral illnesses may impair the metabolism of this drug. They may cause theophylline to be processed either faster or more slowly by the body, causing levels to rise or drop with illness.

Many drugs, such as erythromycin, interact with theophylline. Be certain to tell your child's pediatrician about all medications that you are giving your child, in order to properly balance drug interactions.

TOBRAMYCIN (EYE MEDICATION)

BRAND NAME

Tobradex

GENERAL INFORMATION

Tobramycin is an antibiotic prescribed in eyedrop or ointment form to treat eye infections in children. Eye problems such as conjunctivitis, or pinkeye, are irritating to children and extremely contagious, but prompt treatment will ordinarily clear them up within a day or two.

DOSAGE AND ADMINISTRATION

Tobramycin is available for children as eyedrops or ointment. Apply one to two drops three times a day or ½-inch ribbon of ointment two to three times a day to the affected eye. Ointments are generally easier to apply in young children. Pull down the lower lid and apply the ribbon to the inside of the lower lid.

SIDE EFFECTS

Side effects are uncommon, since tobramycin administered in this manner is not a systemic drug.

IMPORTANT PRECAUTIONS

Tobramycin should be used with caution in children who have demonstrated a previous sensitivity to this type of drug.

TRIAMCINOLONE AND NYSTATIN

BRAND NAMES

Mycolog-II

GENERAL INFORMATION

Mycolog-II is prescribed for the treatment of fungus infections in children. A fungal rash often occurs in the genital area, and appears red, raw, and pimply. Triamcinolone reduces inflammation, while nystatin works by preventing the growth and reproduction of fungus.

DOSAGE AND ADMINISTRATION

Mycolog-II is available topically in cream and ointment form. Apply a thin layer to rash two to four times daily, as directed by your pediatrician.

SIDE EFFECTS

Side effects of treatment with Mycolog-II are uncommon. Local burning or irritation occasionally occurs. If your child experiences these effects, discontinue use and consult your pediatrician.

IMPORTANT PRECAUTIONS

For treatment with Mycolog-II to be effective, it is important to follow the entire course of medication prescribed by your pediatrician. Mycolog-II should not be given to children who have experienced a sensitivity or allergic reaction to it in the past.

TRIAMCINOLONE ACETONIDE

See Corticosteroids, Topical

TRIMETHOPRIM AND SULFAMETHOXAZOLE

BRAND NAMES

Bactrim, Co-Trimazole, Septra

GENERAL INFORMATION

The combination of trimethoprim and sulfamethoxazole, commonly known as Bactrim, is an antibacterial medication prescribed for the treatment of middle ear, upper respiratory, and urinary tract infections in children. The combination of the two drugs in Bactrim is more effective than either one separately in destroying a wide range of bacteria. Bactrim may be an especially effective therapy for ear infections that are amoxicillin-resistant.

Bactrim is only effective against susceptible *bacterial*—not viral, parasitic, or fungal—infections. Your child will usually show signs of improvement following two to five days of treatment. If toxic symptoms or discomfort continue after this time, consult your pediatrician. Your child may be suffering from an infection that is resistant to Bactrim, and another treatment may be more appropriate.

DOSAGE AND ADMINISTRATION

Bactrim is available for children in suspension or tablet form. Children over two months of age should be given Bactrim twice a day for ten to fourteen days. If given as a prophylaxis for urinary tract infections, the dose is one-half the dose given here, only once daily. Doses here are for common respiratory, ear, and urinary tract infections. Your physician may adjust the dosage for children who fall in-between the following weights.

	Suspension	Regular tablets	Double-strength tablets
12 lb	2/3–3/4 tsp*	—	—
22 lb	1–1 1/4 tsp	—	—
33 lb	1 1/2–2 tsp	—	—
44 lb	2–2 1/2 tsp	1	—
66 lb	3–4 tsp	1 1/2–2	—
88 lb	—	2	1

SIDE EFFECTS

The most common side effects of treatment with Bactrim are skin rashes, which usually disappear when treatment is discontinued. Nausea and vomiting are also common reactions. If one or more of these complaints become severe, consult your pediatrician.

While Bactrim is usually well-tolerated, adverse reactions associated with either of its individual components—trimethoprim and sulfamethoxazole—may occur.

Rare but very serious reactions include Stevens-Johnson syndrome (a severe hive-like eruption of the skin associated with inflammation of the membranes of the eyes and mouth), hepatitis (often indicated by severe fatigue and abdominal pain), kidney problems, hypoglycemia blood disorders, and lupus (usually accompanied by a butterfly rash on the face).

Early signs of potentially serious adverse reactions include headache, depression, hallucinations, sore throat, fever, paleness, hives, purple spots on the skin, jaundice, and joint pain. If your child experiences any of these effects, discontinue use at once and consult your pediatrician.

Life-threatening episodes of anaphylaxis (an allergic reaction characterized by sudden respiratory distress, a drop in blood pressure, and the onset of hives) have also been reported. If your child goes into anaphylaxis, call 911 and describe your child's symptoms. Do not try to take your child to the emergency room yourself unless told to do so by emergency personnel. Tell the 911 operator that you need an ambulance immediately.

IMPORTANT PRECAUTIONS

For treatment with Bactrim to be effective—and to prevent infection from recurring—it's important to follow the entire course of medication prescribed by your pediatrician, even after your child's symptoms have diminished or disappeared.

Because it contains a sulfa (sulfonamide) drug, Bactrim should not be given to children under two months of age. It should not be prescribed for children who have experienced a prior sensitivity or allergy to either of its two components. It should be used with caution in children who have impaired liver or kidney function, folic acid deficiency, a history of severe allergies, or asthma.

Children who have G6PD deficiency (mostly children of African or Mediterranean ancestry) should not be given this drug, as it may cause moderately severe anemia over a very few hours.

Since Bactrim may cause heightened light sensitivity, limit your child's exposure to intense sunlight or apply a broad-based sunscreen before going outside.

Many drugs interact with Bactrim. For example, Bactrim may increase the level of phenytoin (Dilantin). Be certain to tell your child's pediatrician about all medications that you are giving your child, in order to properly balance drug interactions.

VALPROIC ACID

BRAND NAMES

Depakene, Depakote

GENERAL INFORMATION

Valproic acid is an anticonvulsant drug prescribed to treat and prevent epileptic seizures in children. This medication may either replace or be used in combination with other anticonvulsant drugs.

However, although valproic acid may be an effective therapy in many cases, it has a number of potential adverse side effects and should be used with caution. Nausea and vomiting occur in over 20 percent of children who are treated with valproic acid. A modification of the drug, divalproex (Depakote), is now used a great deal because it causes much less gastric upset.

DOSAGE AND ADMINISTRATION

Your pediatrician may recommend giving valproic acid to your child with food or medicines to reduce stomach acid if stomach upset is a problem. Divalproex, a modification of valproic acid that results in less stomach distress, has the same dosage guidelines as valproic acid. The medication is available for children in sprinkle, syrup, tablet, and capsule form. It is usually given twice a day, but can be administered one to three times a day with the dose adjusted by simple mathematics.

The dose calculated here is 20 mg per pound per dose. Correct dosage is determined by monitoring blood levels. The initial dose is one-third the dose listed below, and is gradually increased until the drug levels are in the normal range. Your physician may adjust the dosage for children who fall in-between the following weights.

	125 mg sprinkle (Divalproex)	250 mg syrup (Valproic acid)	250 mg tablets/ capsules (Divalproex/ Valproic Acid)	500 mg tablets (Divalproex)
12 lb	1	½ tsp	—	—
22 lb	1–2	1 tsp	—	—
33 lb	2–3	1⅓	—	—
44 lb	3–4	1¾	1–2	—
66 lb	5	2¾	3	—
88 lb	7	3⅔	3–4	1–2

SIDE EFFECTS

Common reactions to valproic acid (Depakote) include gastrointestinal disturbances, especially nausea and vomiting, in almost a quarter of children treated. Diarrhea, stomach cramps, and constipation may also occur occasionally, as well as accompanying changes in appetite and weight. If these problems become severe, speak to your pediatrician about the possibility of replacing valproic acid with divalproex or a different anticonvulsant.

Less common but more serious adverse reactions in children who are given valproic acid are aggressiveness and hyperactivity. More infrequent but potentially serious side effects include headache, tremors, rashes, and alopecia (hair loss).

In rare cases, serious liver damage has been reported. This is usually discovered through blood tests, which must be done regularly during treatment with valproic acid. If your child becomes lethargic and vomits repeatedly, but is otherwise not ill, discontinue treatment at once and consult your pediatrician.

IMPORTANT PRECAUTIONS

Since valproic acid (Depakote) can cause significant side effects in children, careful monitoring by your pediatrician, including regular complete blood counts and liver function testing, is essential.

The discontinuation of treatment with valproic acid should be accomplished on a gradual basis, according to the exact instructions of your pediatrician, so as not to aggravate seizures.

Many drugs interact with valproic acid. When the two anticonvulsants valproic acid and phenytoin are prescribed together, the effect is complex; the level of valproic acid in the body can be either increased or decreased through interaction with phenytoin (Dilantin). Other drugs that may interact with valproic acid include phenobarbital and carbamazepine (Tegretol).

Be certain to tell your child's pediatrician about all medications that you are giving your child, in order to properly balance drug interactions.

6

BASIC OVER-THE-COUNTER MEDICATIONS FOR CHILDREN

In this chapter you will find an accessible and easy-to-use A-to-Z guide to the over-the-counter medications most commonly used for children. As in Chapter Five, where we discussed prescription drugs, over-the-counter products are alphabetized by their generic name, which is the same as their primary active ingredient. Below this, we list brand names with which you may be familiar. If you want to look up a product by brand name, just turn to the product index.

In addition, in each profile you will find:

- General information about the medication
- What type of dosage is appropriate for your child
- How to best administer the medication
- How often to administer the medication
- What common side effects to keep an eye out for

- More serious adverse reactions that may warrant discontinuing the medication and consulting your pediatrician
- Important precautions, such as drug interactions

While individual profiles also include some ingredients used in cold remedies, we conclude our chapter with an in-depth look at cough and cold preparations, the over-the-counter remedies most commonly used in children. The differences among these remedies are minimal, yet most parents want to know whether the medications they are giving their children contain dye or alcohol. Frequency of dosing is also an issue. We examine the many different components of these medications, discuss the pros and cons of combination drugs, and conclude with a handy table characterizing thirty of the most frequently used products. Parents can compare products and choose the one that best fits their child's needs.

Over-the-Counter Medications

Acetaminophen
Aspirin
Bisacodyl
Charcoal, Activated
Chlorpheniramine Maleate
Clotrimazole
Dextromethorphan
Dimenhydrinate
Diphenhydramine
Guaifenesin
Hydrocortisone
Ibuprofen
Ipecac
Iron
Loperamide
Magnesium Hydroxide
Miconazole
Permethrin
Phenylephrine
Pseudoephedrine
Pyrethins
Selenium Sulfide
Tolnaftate

ACETAMINOPHEN

BRAND NAMES

Liquiprin, Panadol, Tempra, Tylenol

GENERAL INFORMATION

Aspirin-free acetaminophen provides fast, effective relief for children's pain and fever. Cases in which acetaminophen may be appropriate include discomfort due to colds and flu, teething, immunizations, and injury. Acetaminophen does not interact with ibuprofen or other regularly used symptom-relief medications.

In the majority of cases, children should be given acetaminophen in place of aspirin. Children who are given aspirin, especially when they have chicken pox, flu, or flulike symptoms, may develop a life-threatening condition called Reye syndrome. The symptoms of Reye syndrome usually occur toward the end of the original illness, and may include extreme tiredness, violent headache, disorientation, belligerence, and vomiting.

DOSAGE AND ADMINISTRATION

Most children enjoy the taste of acetaminophen, so administration is not generally difficult. Acetaminophen is available for children as infant drops, elixir, chewable tablets, and junior caplets or chewables. It is given every four hours, up to five doses in twenty-four hours.

Dosages may be adjusted for children who fall in-between the following weights. Your pediatrician may recommend the higher dosage ranges of acetaminophen when your child is suffering from a very high fever.

	Infant drops	Elixir	Chewable tablets (80mg)	Junior caplets or chewables (160 mg)
12 lb	0.8 cc (1 dropperful)	½ tsp	—	—
22 lb	1.0–1.5 cc (1¼–2 droppersful)	¾–1 tsp	1–2	—
33 lb	1.5–2.25 cc (2–3 droppersful)	1–1½ tsp	2–3	1
44 lb	—	1¼–2 tsp	2–4	1–2
66 lb	—	2–2¾ tsp	4–6	2–3
88 lb	—	2½–3¾ tsp	—	3–4

SIDE EFFECTS

No side effects are associated with acetaminophen when suggested dosages are correctly administered.

Prolonged use of large doses of acetaminophen may cause kidney or liver problems, especially damage to these organs; these are very rare in otherwise healthy children. Symptoms include nausea and vomiting.

IMPORTANT PRECAUTIONS

Consult your pediatrician if fever persists for more than three days or if pain continues for more than five days.

ASPIRIN

BRAND NAMES

Bayer, St. Joseph's

WARNING:

Children who are given aspirin, especially when they have chicken pox, flu, or flulike symptoms, may develop a life-threatening condition called Reye syndrome. The symptoms of Reye syndrome usually occur toward the end of the original illness, and may include extreme tiredness, violent headache, disorientation, belligerence, and vomiting.

GENERAL INFORMATION

Aspirin was once the most important drug for fever, pain, and inflammation in children. However, with the recognition of Reye syndrome in children, aspirin is no longer used except in special circumstances, such as arthritis, rheumatic fever, and Kawasaki disease (an illness characterized by high fever and inflamed mucous membranes, which can cause damage to heart vessels), where the benefits outweigh the risks.

Other drugs, such as acetaminophen, are as effective and much safer than aspirin for fever and pain. Ibuprofen has the same effects as aspirin for fever, pain, and inflammation, but does not cause Reye syndrome.

DOSAGE AND ADMINISTRATION

Aspirin should be given to children only under close medical supervision. Dosage is tailored to the specific problem, and is often monitored with blood tests when given in high doses.

SIDE EFFECTS

The most common side effects of aspirin are heartburn and upset stomach in individuals who are sensitive to it. Fortunately, this is less likely in children than adults.

Less common adverse reactions to aspirin include allergic reactions such as skin rashes, liver toxicity, and decreased coagulation of blood. High doses may cause ringing in the ears, which usually resolves when the dose is lowered.

IMPORTANT PRECAUTIONS

Do not give aspirin to children who have fever and discomfort with viral illness, especially chicken pox and influenza. This can put children at risk of the serious and potentially life-threatening condition, Reye syndrome. Children who are given aspirin should be carefully monitored by their pediatrician. Interestingly, however, children receiving aspirin chronically seem to be at little or no risk of Reye syndrome.

BISACODYL

BRAND NAME

Dulcolax

GENERAL INFORMATION:

Bisacodyl is a laxative used to treat constipation in children. This drug acts on the smooth muscles of the intestine wall to stimulate bowel movement. A bowel movement usually occurs six hours after oral administration, and fifteen minutes after rectal insertion. Bisacodyl is generally not recommended for children under six years of age.

DOSAGE AND ADMINISTRATION

Bisacodyl is available for children as tablets or suppositories. The tablets should not be chewed or crushed. Oral bisacodyl is given six hours before the desired bowel movement; suppositories give prompt results. Dosages may be adjusted for children who fall in-between the following weights.

	5 mg tab & suppository	10 mg suppository
12 lb	Bisacodyl is not recommended for this group.	
22 lb		
33 lb		
44 lb	1	—
66 lb	1–2	1
88 lb	1–3	1

SIDE EFFECTS

A common side effect of treatment with bisacodyl is rectal irritation. If this complaint becomes severe, consult your pediatrician.

Less frequent adverse reactions to bisacodyl include cramps, nausea, and potassium deficiency. In rare cases, irritability, headache, confusion, difficulty breathing, irregular heartbeat, muscle cramps, and unusual tiredness may develop. If your child experiences any of these effects, discontinue use and consult your pediatrician.

IMPORTANT PRECAUTIONS

Bisacodyl should not be given to children within one hour of other medications, since laxatives may interfere with their absorption.

Bisacodyl should be used with caution in children who have congestive heart failure, diabetes, or high blood pressure.

Other drugs, such as cimetidine, ranitidine, and antacids, interact with bisacodyl. Consult with your pediatrician if your child is taking other medications in addition to bisacodyl.

CHARCOAL, ACTIVATED

BRAND NAMES

Acta-Char, Actidose-Aqua, Aqueous Charcodote, Charcoaid, Charcocaps, Charcodote, Insta-Char, Liqui-Char, SuperChar

WARNING

Under no circumstances should you administer activated charcoal without first consulting your poison center or pediatrician.

GENERAL INFORMATION

Activated charcoal, along with ipecac, is used for the treatment of poisonings from medication or other substances. Activated charcoal is a powder that is mixed with water. It should always be kept in your emergency first-aid kit. Activated charcoal helps prevent poison from being absorbed from the stomach and intestines.

DOSAGE AND ADMINISTRATION

Administer activated charcoal to your child only as directed by your pediatrician or poison control center. Since the average patient who ingests activated charcoal is eighteen to twenty-four months old, and the charcoal is black, gritty, and odd- (although not bad-) tasting, they spit it out or vomit it up. This helps remove the poison. Use a straw to give the mixture to your child, and be prepared to mop and wipe up the mess afterwards.

SIDE EFFECTS

A common side effect to the administration of activated charcoal is black bowel movements.

No serious adverse reactions occur from the use of activated charcoal. In rare cases, however, constipation occurs. A laxative should be given to remedy this condition.

IMPORTANT PRECAUTIONS

Always consult your pediatrician or poison control center before giving antidotes to poison to your child. Activated charcoal should not be administered in cases where the poison ingested was lye, strong acids, cyanide, iron, ethyl alcohol, or methyl alcohol.

Activated charcoal should not be given with other medications or food, which may decrease its absorption.

Note: Your poison control center is listed in your phone book, usually in the front with other numbers. If it is not, any operator can assist you. Also, see ipecac.

CHLORPHENIRAMINE MALEATE

BRANDS THAT CONTAIN THIS DRUG

Chlortrimeton, Novahistine, PediaCare Cough Cold, PediaCare Night Rest, Robitussin Pediatric Night Relief, Triaminic Nite Lite Triaminic Syrup, Triaminicol, Trind, Trind DM, Tylenol Cold, Vicks DaQuil, Vicks Nyquil

GENERAL INFORMATION

Chlorpheniramine maleate is an antihistamine used in many allergy, cold, and cough preparations. This drug blocks the effect of histamine, a substance released in allergic reactions such as itching and inflammation. In the treatment of allergies, chlorpheniramine works by drying the membranes and thus drying up runny noses. Many colds will not respond to antihistamines, and the effect of the drug varies from child to child. Chlorpheniramine is by far the most popular antihistamine on the market today.

DOSAGE AND ADMINISTRATION

Chlorpheniramine is given every four to six hours, up to four times daily. Dosages may be adjusted for children who fall in-between the following ages.

	Syrup	Chewable tablets	4mg tablets
Under 2	Not recommended under age 2.		
2–6 Yrs.	½	½	—
6–12 Yrs.	1	1	½–1

SIDE EFFECTS

The most common side effect of treatment with chlorpheniramine is drowsiness.

An occasional adverse reaction to chlorpheniramine in very young children is hyperactivity for a few hours. *Less frequent adverse reactions* include dizziness, dry mouth and throat, and nausea. If your child experiences any of these effects, discontinue use and consult your pediatrician.

IMPORTANT PRECAUTIONS

Chlorpheniramine is not an appropriate medication for children who have glaucoma or kidney disease.

Be sure to consult with your pediatrician if your child is taking other medications in addition to chlorpheniramine, so that possible drug interactions can be balanced.

CLOTRIMAZOLE

BRAND NAMES

Cruex, Desenex, Lotrimin

GENERAL INFORMATION

Clotrimazole is an antifungal medication recommended to treat a whitish fungal condition in the mouth known as thrush, and other fungal infections, such as diaper rash and certain other skin rashes. Clotrimazole works by interfering with the permeability of the fungal cell wall, thereby killing it.

DOSAGE AND ADMINISTRATION

Clotrimazole is available for children in cream, lotion, or solution form. A small amount should be applied to the affected area twice daily for three to five days. The dosage is the same for all ages.

SIDE EFFECTS

Side effects to treatment with clotrimazole are uncommon. Infrequent adverse reactions include redness, burning, itching, and inflammation at the site of application. If your child experiences any of these effects, discontinue use and consult your pediatrician.

IMPORTANT PRECAUTIONS

Wash your hands before and after applying clotrimazole. Avoid the eye area.

Clotrimazole should be used for the full period of recommended treatment. Consult your pediatrician if symptoms have not cleared up by this time.

DEXTROMETHORPHAN

BRANDS THAT CONTAIN THIS DRUG

Benylin-DM, Children's Nyquil Nighttime Cold Medicine, Contac Jr. Children's Cold Medicine, PediaCare, Robitussin-DM, Triaminic-DM

GENERAL INFORMATION

Dextromethorphan is the cough suppressant in all the over-the-counter cold and cough preparations. Dextromethorphan suppresses the urge to cough. It works by reducing the sensitivity of the brain's cough control center. It is an excellent drug because it will not suppress a necessary cough or keep a child from clearing out excess secretions.

DOSAGE AND ADMINISTRATION

Dextromethorphan is available for children in a wide variety of cold and cough preparations as syrup, tablets, and lozenges.

Administer remedies that contain dextromethorphan to your child according to label instructions, since each brand has different concentrations, doses, and frequencies of administration. Use measuring spoons or droppers to accurately measure medication, and discontinue medication when symptoms disappear.

SIDE EFFECTS

There are *no minor, frequently occurring* side effects due to treatment with dextromethorphan.

Infrequent adverse reactions are confusion, excitement, and nervousness. More rarely, dizziness, drowsiness, rash, diarrhea, nausea, and vomiting have been reported. If your child experiences any of these effects, discontinue use and consult your pediatrician.

IMPORTANT PRECAUTIONS

Dextromethorphan may not be an appropriate medication for children who suffer from liver problems.

If cough persists for four days or more, if your child coughs up blood, or if your child does not respond to this cough suppressant, consult your pediatrician.

Prolonged use of dextromethorphan may lead to dependence.

Be sure to consult with your pediatrician if your child is taking other medications in addition to dextromethorphan, so that possible drug interactions can be balanced.

DIMENHYDRINATE

BRAND NAME

Dramamine

GENERAL INFORMATION

Dimenhydrinate is used to prevent and treat motion sickness in children. Some children experience nausea, vomiting, and dizziness due to the motion of cars, boats, planes, or trains, as the semicircular canal in the ear is affected and equilibrium is disturbed. For reasons that remain unclear, dimenhydrinate restores this equilibrium.

DOSAGE AND ADMINISTRATION

Dimenhydrinate is available for children as tablets, chewable tablets, and in liquid form, and should be given one hour before travel time and repeated every six hours as needed. Dosages may be adjusted for children who fall in-between the following weights.

	16 mg/5 ml solution	50 mg chewable
12 lb	1/3 tsp	—
22 lb	3/4 tsp	1/4
33 lb	1 1/4 tsp	1/3
44 lb	1 1/2 tsp	1/2
66 lb	2 1/3 tsp	3/4
88 lb	—	1

SIDE EFFECTS

The most common side effect from treatment with dimenhydrinate is drowsiness. Your child may also experience dry mouth and throat.

An occasional more serious side effect is blurred vision. If this occurs, discontinue medication and consult your pediatrician.

IMPORTANT PRECAUTIONS

Be sure to consult with your pediatrician if your child is taking other medications, such as antibiotics, so that possible drug interactions can be balanced.

DIPHENHYDRAMINE

BRAND NAMES

Benadryl Decongestant Elixir, Benadryl Elixir

GENERAL INFORMATION

Diphenhydramine is a mild antihistamine that is used in many cold and cough remedies to relieve allergic symptoms. It also has a calming, sedative effect. Diphenhydramine is helpful in many types of allergies, including hay fever, hives, and rashes. It works by blocking the action of histamine after an allergic response has triggered it.

DOSAGE AND ADMINISTRATION

Diphenhydramine should be administered one hour before or two hours after meals. It is given four times a day, every six hours. Higher doses should be used for hives and sedation.

Diphenhydramine is available for children in liquid or tablet form. Dosages may be adjusted for children who fall in-between the following weights.

	12.5 mg syrup	25 mg tablets or capsules	50 mg tablets or capsules
12 lb	½ tsp	—	—
22 lb	1 tsp	—	—
33 lb	1½ tsp	—	—
44 lb	2 tsp	1	—
66 lb	3 tsp	1	—
88 lb	—	2	1

SIDE EFFECTS

The most common side effect of treatment with diphenhydramine is sleepiness. Young children under age three can have a paradoxical reaction and become very active when taking diphenhydramine. Discontinue the drug if this occurs.

Less frequent or adverse reactions include dizziness, dry mouth and throat, and nausea. If your child experiences any of these effects, discontinue use and consult your pediatrician.

IMPORTANT PRECAUTIONS

Diphenhydramine is not an appropriate medication for children who have asthma, glaucoma, or kidney disease. Medications containing diphenhydramine should be given with caution to children who are scheduled for surgery in the next two months.

Be sure to consult with your pediatrician if your child is taking other medications in addition to diphenhydramine, so that possible drug interactions can be balanced.

GUAIFENESIN

BRANDS THAT CONTAIN THIS DRUG

Benylin Expectorant, Entuss Pediatric Expectorant, Naldecon-DX, Nucofed Pediatric Expectorant, Robitussin, Triaminic Expectorant, Vicks Children's Cough

GENERAL INFORMATION

Guaifenesin is an ingredient in many cold and cough preparations. Guaifenesin loosens excess mucus in respiratory passages due to allergies or infections. It works by increasing the production of watery fluids to dilute thin mucus so that it can be coughed out or absorbed. Its effectiveness is not well-proven.

DOSAGE AND ADMINISTRATION

Guaifenesin is available for children in a wide variety of cold and cough preparations as syrup, drops, tablets, and capsules.

Administer remedies that contain guaifenesin to your child as directed and when needed, but not more often than every four hours. Carefully read and follow the directions on the label. Use measuring spoons or droppers to accurately measure medication, and discontinue medication when symptoms disappear.

SIDE EFFECTS

No minor side effects commonly occur from treatment with guaifenesin.

Infrequent serious side effects or adverse reactions are rash, stomachache, diarrhea, nausea, and vomiting. If your child experiences any of these effects, discontinue use and consult your pediatrician.

IMPORTANT PRECAUTIONS

None.

HYDROCORTISONE

BRAND NAMES

CaldeCORT, Clinicort, Cortaid, Cortif, Hycort

GENERAL INFORMATION

Hydrocortisone is a mild topical anti-inflammatory corticosteroid used to relieve skin rashes in children. These itchy, irritating, and often oozing rashes include eczema, contact dermatitis (a rash due to contact with irritants ranging from poison ivy to detergents used to wash clothing to nickel in jewelry), and psoriasis.

While the exact causes of most rashes remain unknown, certain children appear especially prone to developing them, probably due to genetic predisposition. Identifying and avoiding the substance or substances that trigger rashes is important, as is keeping your child's fingernails well-clipped when rashes develop.

Depending on the severity of the rash, you may require hydrocortisone in ½ to 1 percent strength. If over-the-counter products alone do not control the rash, your pediatrician will prescribe a stronger topical corticosteroid, such as fluocinonide or betamethasone. (For a comprehensive discussion of topical corticosteroids, turn to page 102.)

DOSAGE AND ADMINISTRATION

Hydrocortisone is available in cream, lotion, ointment, and spray form. Apply twice daily. A thin film is sufficient, and treated skin should ideally be left exposed to the air, or at most, loosely covered. Never cover with tight bandages unless specifically directed by your doctor.

SIDE EFFECTS

The most common side effect of treatment with hydrocortisone is skin irritation and dryness. To avoid these problems, use the smallest effective amount.

Less common adverse reactions are burning, itching, and severe skin irritation.

If your child experiences any of these effects, discontinue use at once and consult your pediatrician.

IMPORTANT PRECAUTIONS

Hydrocortisone should be used sparingly and for short periods of time (approximately one week) in order to minimize the risk of side effects. Hydrocortisone is for external use only. Do not apply it in the sensitive area around your child's eyes.

IBUPROFEN

BRAND NAMES

Advil or Motrin for Children

GENERAL INFORMATION

Ibuprofen is now an over-the-counter medication for children as well as adults. Like acetaminophen, aspirin-free ibuprofen is an effective way of reducing fever in children. It is also a helpful anti-inflammatory agent. Ibuprofen works by reducing the concentration of prostaglandins (hormones that can lead to pain and inflammation) in tissues.

Children should generally be given ibuprofen or acetaminophen instead of aspirin. Aspirin in children, especially when they have chicken pox, flu, or flulike symptoms, has been associated with a life-threatening condition called Reye syndrome. Reye syndrome does not occur with ibuprofen. Ibuprofen has no interaction with acetaminophen.

DOSAGE AND ADMINISTRATION

Ibuprofen is available for children in suspension and tablet form. The dose of ibuprofen is unusual, because the dose depends on the level of the child's fever. In this table, dosages are arranged by the child's temperature, rather than the

	Temp. ≤ 102° F.	Temp. > 102° F.
12 lb	Not approved < 6 months	
22 lb	½ tsp suspension	1 tsp suspension
33 lb	¾ tsp suspension	1½ tsp suspension
44 lb	1 tsp suspension or 1 chewable tablet	2 tsp suspension or 2 chewable tablets
66 lb	1½ tsp suspension	3 tsp suspension
88 lb	2 tsp suspension or 1 chewable tablet	4 tsp suspension or 4 chewable tablets

form of the medication. Ibuprofen may be given every six hours as needed. Dosages may be adjusted for children who fall in-between the weights in the chart on page 221.

SIDE EFFECTS

Common side effects of treatment with ibuprofen are intestinal distress, such as nausea and heartburn. While this is a problem with adults, it has occurred much less frequently in children.

Infrequent adverse reactions are muscle cramps, numbness, and difficulty breathing. Long-term use of ibuprofen can lead to eye damage, reduced hearing, and a suppression of certain blood cells that fight infection. If your child experiences any of these effects, discontinue use and consult your pediatrician.

IMPORTANT PRECAUTIONS

Ibuprofen is not an appropriate remedy for children who suffer from kidney or liver problems. It should be used with caution in children who have ulcers, gastritis, asthma, high blood pressure, or breathing problems, or who are known to be sensitive to aspirin, naprosyn, or other similar drugs.

Be sure to consult with your pediatrician if your child is taking other medications in addition to ibuprofen, so that possible drug interactions can be balanced.

IPECAC

WARNING

Under no circumstances should you give ipecac to your child without first consulting your poison center or pediatrician.

GENERAL INFORMATION

Ipecac is used for the treatment of medication overdose and in some cases of poisoning. It should always be kept in your emergency first-aid kit. Ipecac works by irritating the stomach lining and stimulating the vomiting center in the brain. Today ipecac is used less often than activated charcoal in treating cases of poisoning.

DOSAGE AND ADMINISTRATION

Administer ipecac to your child only as directed by your pediatrician or poison control center. The child should be sufficiently alert to sit up and vomit into a basin.

SIDE EFFECTS

Ipecac is intended to make your child vomit, so a certain amount of discomfort can be anticipated.

An irregular heartbeat is a very rare but life-threatening adverse reaction to ipecac. Immediate emergency treatment is required.

IMPORTANT PRECAUTIONS

Always consult your pediatrician or poison control center before giving antidotes to poison to your child. Ipecac should not be administered in cases where the poison ingested was a corrosive substance, such as acid, bleach, cleaning fluid, furniture polish, gasoline, kerosene, or lye.

Ipecac should not be given with other medications, which may decrease its absorption.

If you are instructed to give your child activated charcoal as well as ipecac, administer charcoal after vomiting induced by ipecac. Activated charcoal is best given in an emergency room.

Note: Your poison control center is listed in your phone book, usually in the front with other numbers. If it is not, any operator can assist you. Also, see Charcoal, activated.

IRON

BRAND NAMES

Feosol, Feostat, Fergon, Fer-In-Sol, Fer-Iron, Fero-Grad, Ferralet, Ferralyn, Ferrospace

GENERAL INFORMATION

Iron supplements are recommended for children who have a dietary iron deficiency or iron-deficiency anemia. Since poor eating habits are often the cause of iron deficiencies, incorporating plenty of iron-rich foods into your child's diet is helpful. Meat, poultry, fish, beans, leafy green vegetables, and fortified cereals are rich sources of iron. Iron supplements stimulate the bone marrow's production of hemoglobin, the red blood cell pigment that carries oxygen to cells throughout the body.

DOSAGE AND ADMINISTRATION

Iron supplements should not be given with beverages or food, which will decrease absorption. Liquid iron can be mixed with water or juice to avoid temporary tooth discoloration.

The dosages and forms of iron are not standardized. Iron tablets may be 195-mg, 300-mg, and 324-mg or 250-mg capsules. The table below illustrates a representative sample. Brand names are used here because there is a wide variation between forms. These brands account for most forms of iron dispensed for children. Ferrous sulfate is the usual form of iron prescribed and is the active ingredient in Fer-In-Sol and Feosol. Ferrous gluconate is sometimes used.

Doses in brackets [ ] are for daily supplement dosage; this dosage is given once daily. This dosage is followed by dosages for mild, then moderate or severe iron deficiency anemia; this dose is given twice daily. Dosages may be adjusted for children who fall in-between the following weights.

	Fer-In-Sol drops (15 mg iron/ 0.6cc dropper)	Fer-In-Sol Syrup (18 mg iron/tsp)	Feosol elixir (44 mg iron/ tsp)	Ferrous sulfate tablets—300 mg (60 mg elemental iron)	Ferrous gluconate elixir (34 mg elemental iron/tsp) (7% alcohol)	Ferrous gluconate tablets—300 mg (34 mg elemental iron/tsp)
12 lb	[0.3cc] 0.3/0.6cc	—	—	—	—	—
22 lb	[0.6cc] 0.6/1.2cc	[1 tsp] 1–2 tsp	—	—	—	—
33 lb	[0.6cc] 0.9/1.8cc	[1 tsp] 1½–3 tsp	[—] ½–1 tsp	—	—	—
44 lb	—	[⅔ tsp]	[—] ⅔–1½ tsp	—	[—] 1–2 tsp	—
66 lb	—	[⅔ tsp]	[—] 1–2 tsp	—	[—] 1½–3 tsp	—
88 lb	—	[⅔ tsp]	[—] 1½–3 tsp	[—] 1 tablet 2 or 3 times daily	[—] 3–6 tsp	2 tablets 2 or 3 times daily

SIDE EFFECTS

Common side effects of treatment with iron supplements are black or gray stools. Stained teeth may result from the use of liquid iron.

Less frequent adverse reactions include stomach pain, constipation or diarrhea, heartburn, nausea, and vomiting. If your child experiences any of these effects, discontinue use and consult your pediatrician. A lower dose may be necessary to prevent side effects.

IMPORTANT PRECAUTIONS

Iron tablets look like sugar-coated candy. They should not be given to younger children because of the potential for them to ingest extra medication, resulting in poisoning. It is especially important to store iron pills safely and securely in childproof containers.

Iron supplements are not an appropriate medication for children who have acute hepatitis or hemolytic anemia. They should be used with caution in children who have a peptic ulcer, enteritis, or colitis.

It's important not to exceed the recommended dosage of iron supplements. An overdose of iron can be serious, with symptoms ranging from vomiting and weakened pulse to lowered blood pressure and internal bleeding.

Iron supplements may decrease the concentration of drugs such as tetracycline, while medications such as antacids may decrease the effect of iron. Be certain to tell your child's pediatrician about all medications that you are giving your child, in order to properly balance drug interactions.

LOPERAMIDE

BRAND NAMES

Imodium, Imodium A-D, Pepto-Bismol for Diarrhea

GENERAL INFORMATION

Loperamide is recommended to relieve diarrhea in children. It works by reducing irritability and contractions in the intestinal tract, and should be effective within one to two hours of administration. If severe diarrhea lasts more than twenty-four hours, consult your pediatrician.

DOSAGE AND ADMINISTRATION

Loperamide is available in liquid, tablet, and capsule form for children. It should not be used for children under two, and a manufacturer suggests a pediatrician be consulted before giving to children under six.

Loperamide should be given at the first diarrheal stool. If diarrhea continues, the dose can be repeated as a half-dose up to the maximum stated below. However, often a single dose is effective. Dosages may be adjusted for children who fall in-between the following weights.

	1 mg/tsp liquid	2 mg tablet/capsule
12 lb	Not to be used under 2 years of age.	
22 lb	1 tsp, then ½ tsp × 2 max	—
33 lb	1 tsp, then ½ tsp × 2 max	—
44 lb	2 tsp, then 1 tsp × 2 max	—
66 lb	2 tsp, then 1 tsp × 4 max	—
88 lb	4 tsp, then 2 tsp × 2 max	2 tab/cap, then 1 × 2 max

SIDE EFFECTS

Minor side effects from treatment with loperamide are rare.

Less frequent adverse reactions include dizziness, stomach pain, constipation, bloating, and loss of appetite. If your child experiences any of these effects, discontinue use and consult your pediatrician.

IMPORTANT PRECAUTIONS

Loperamide should not be given to children who suffer from colitis.

It is important to inform your pediatrician at once if your child appears dehydrated due to fluid loss from diarrhea.

If your child has a fever of 102 degrees or higher, or if stools are bloody, consult your pediatrician before using loperamide.

MAGNESIUM HYDROXIDE

BRAND NAME

Phillips' Milk of Magnesia

GENERAL INFORMATION

Magnesium hydroxide is a gentle laxative used to treat constipation in children. This drug helps loosen stools and move them out of your child's intestine. To prevent or cure constipation, you can also make sure that your child takes plenty of fluids and follows a diet rich in fiber. Leafy green vegetables, prunes, and whole grains are helpful.

DOSAGE AND ADMINISTRATION

Magnesium hydroxide is available for children as an oral suspension. Since this medication may have a slightly disagreeable chalky taste, try diluting it in a small glass of water or juice. Milk of Magnesia is given when needed. When administered one half-hour after meals and at bedtime, it will prevent acid rebound after meals and hyperacidity at night. Dosages may be adjusted for children who fall in-between the following weights.

	Suspension
12 lb	rarely used
22 lb	1 tsp
33 lb	1½ tsp
44 lb	2 tsp
66 lb	3 tsp
88 lb	4 tsp

SIDE EFFECTS

Frequently occurring side effects due to treatment with magnesium hydroxide are relatively uncommon.

Large amounts of magnesium hydroxide may cause diarrhea. It can also cause low blood pressure and suppress respiration when given in high doses for long periods of time.

If your child experiences any ill effects while taking magnesium hydroxide, discontinue use and consult your pediatrician.

IMPORTANT PRECAUTIONS

Magnesium hydroxide should be used with caution in children who have stomach pain, nausea, vomiting, chronic constipation, colitis, or symptoms of appendicitis.

Consult your pediatrician before giving magnesium hydroxide to a child who has kidney disease.

Laxatives should not be given for prolonged periods of time, since habitual use may create dependence and impair the body's natural process of waste removal.

Be sure to speak to your pediatrician if your child is taking other medications in addition to magnesium hydroxide, so that possible drug interactions can be balanced.

MICONAZOLE

BRAND NAMES

Monistat, Mycelex, Mycostatin

GENERAL INFORMATION

Miconazole is an antifungal medication recommended to treat a variety of fungal infections, such as diaper rash, athlete's foot, ringworm, and nail fungus. It works by damaging fungal cell walls. Miconazole must generally be used for two to eight weeks to be effective.

DOSAGE AND ADMINISTRATION

Miconazole is available for children as a cream, lotion, ointment, gel, or powder. Apply small amounts to affected areas twice daily. When possible, leave treated areas exposed to air. Miconazole is also available as a shampoo, which should be used once a day.

SIDE EFFECTS

Frequently occurring side effects to treatment with miconazole are uncommon.

Infrequent adverse reactions include itching, redness, and inflammation at the site of application. If your child experiences any of these effects, discontinue use and consult your pediatrician.

IMPORTANT PRECAUTIONS

Miconazole should not be used with other skin medications, unless directed by your pediatrician.

Wash your hands before and after applying miconazole. Avoid the eye area.

PERMETHRIN

BRAND NAMES

Nix Creme Rinse, Prioderm, Pronto Lice Killing Shampoo

GENERAL INFORMATION

Permethrin is used to treat lice infestations of the scalp. If there is a lice outbreak at your child's day care center, school, or camp, you must check your child's scalp every day, morning and evening, for seven days. Children are in frequent physical contact with one another, so head lice are very likely to pass from one child to the next.

To detect head lice, look for small white eggs (nits) that look like dandruff attached to the hair shaft and are located at the base of your child's scalp. If you find one, try to remove it from the hair shaft with your fingernails. If it doesn't come off, it is lice.

In addition to washing or rinsing your child's hair with medication, you will need to launder your child's clothing, towels, and bedding in the hot water cycle. Combs and brushes should be dropped in boiling water for one minute to disinfect them. Hats and head gear should be washed, drycleaned or put in a plastic bag for two weeks. Lice can otherwise persist in children's environments and reinfect them.

DOSAGE AND ADMINISTRATION

Thoroughly wash or rinse your child's hair with shampoo, rinse, and towel dry. Apply a sufficient volume of a permethrin product to saturate the hair and scalp. Leave on for ten minutes, and then rinse thoroughly. One thorough washing or rinse should be sufficient, as long as you are also certain to take appropriate measures to remove all lice from your child's environment. Permethrin also has a residual effect that lasts for several weeks.

SIDE EFFECTS

Side effects with permethrin are limited to allergic skin rashes, primarily in children with sensitive skin. If your child develops a skin rash after treatment with permethrin, consult your pediatrician.

IMPORTANT PRECAUTIONS

Permethrin is not for internal use. If your child accidentally swallows this product, call your poison control center. Permethrin should not be applied on open sores or wounds. If your child is prone to allergic reactions of the skin such as eczema, consult your pediatrician before using.

Protect your child's eyes from exposure to this product.

If the eyes are accidentally exposed, immediately flush them with plenty of cold water.

Use plastic gloves to apply the shampoo, and open the bathroom window to make sure the room is well-ventilated. Avoid inhaling permethrin fumes.

PHENYLEPHRINE

BRANDS WHICH CONTAIN THIS DRUG

Dimetane, Dimetapp, Naldecon Pediatric, Novahistine, Phenergan VC, Robitussin Night Relief

GENERAL INFORMATION

Phenylephrine is an ingredient in many cold and cough preparations. Phenylephrine reduces congestion of the nose, sinuses, and throat due to allergies or infections. It works by decreasing blood volume in nasal tissues, shrinking swollen membranes, and opening blocked airways.

DOSAGE AND ADMINISTRATION

Phenylephrine is avilable for children as syrup, drops, tablets, and capsules in a wide variety of cold and cough preparations.

Administer remedies that contain phenylephrine to your child as directed and when needed, but no more often than every four hours. Carefully read and follow the directions on the label. Use measuring spoons or droppers to accurately measure medication, and discontinue medication when symptoms disappear.

SIDE EFFECTS

A common side effect of treatment with phenylephrine is a fast or pounding heartbeat. This is not a serious problem.

Less common serious side effects or adverse reactions include headache, dizziness, insomnia, nervousness, and dryness in the nose. If your child experiences any of these effects, discontinue use and consult your pediatrician.

IMPORTANT PRECAUTIONS

Phenylephrine should be used with caution in children who have high blood pressure, heart disease, diabetes, or thyroid problems. Prolonged use of decongestants such as phenylephrine can result in a rebound effect, in which the body becomes dependent on the drug, losing the normal ability to fight congestion and requiring ever greater amounts of decongestant to have an impact.

PSEUDOEPHEDRINE

BRANDS WHICH CONTAIN THIS DRUG

Benadryl, Benylin Decongestant, Children's Nyquil, Children's Sudafed Liquid, Dorcol Children's Cold Formula, Drixoral, Nucofed Pediatric Expectorant, PediaCare, Robitussin-PE, Triaminic Nite Light

GENERAL INFORMATION

Pseudoephedrine is an ingredient in many cold and cough preparations. Pseudoephedrine reduces congestion of the nose, sinuses, and throat due to allergies or infections. It works by decreasing blood volume in nasal tissues, shrinking swollen membranes, and opening blocked airways.

DOSAGE AND ADMINISTRATION

Pseudoephedrine is available for children as drops, syrup, or tablets. It is given every six hours as needed. Pseudoephedrine is also a component of many decongestant remedies, often at a lower dose.

	7.5 mg/.8ml drops	15 mg/tsp syrup	30 mg/tsp syrup	30 mg tablets
12 lb	0.6 cc*	—	—	—
22 lb	1.0 cc*	—	—	—
33 lb	—	1 tsp	½ tsp	—
44 lb	—	1⅓ tsp	⅔ tsp	—
66 lb	—	2 tsp	1 tsp	1
88 lb	—	—	1 tsp	1

SIDE EFFECTS

The most common side effects of treatment with pseudoephedrine are agitation, irritability, and insomnia. If one or more of these complaints become severe, consult your pediatrician.

Less frequent adverse reactions include nausea, vomiting, a change in heartbeat, difficulty in breathing, painful urination, sweating, and trembling. If your child experiences any of these effects, discontinue use and consult your pediatrician.

IMPORTANT PRECAUTIONS

Pseudoephedrine should be used with caution in young infants, as hyperirritability is a common side effect.

Pseudoephedrine is not an appropriate medication for children who have an overactive thyroid condition, diabetes, high blood pressure, or heart disease.

Be sure to consult with your pediatrician if your child is taking other medications in addition to pseudoephedrine, so that possible drug interactions can be balanced.

PYRETHINS

BRAND NAMES

A-200, Pyrinyl, R&C, RID, Scabene, Thionex, Triple X

GENERAL INFORMATION

Pyrethins are formulated into shampoos to treat lice infestations of the scalp. If there is a lice outbreak at your child's day care center, school, or camp, you must check your child's scalp every day, morning and evening, for seven days. Children are in frequent physical contact with one another, so head lice are very likely to pass from one child to the next.

To detect head lice, look for small white eggs (nits) that look like dandruff attached to the hair shaft, and are located at the base of your child's scalp. If you find one, try to remove it from the hair shaft with your fingernails. If it doesn't come off readily, the nits indicate a head lice infestation.

In addition to washing or rinsing your child's hair with medication, you will need to launder your child's clothing, towels, and bedding in the hot water cycle. Combs and brushes should be dropped in boiling water for one minute to disinfect them. Hats and head gear should be washed, drycleaned or put in a plastic bag for two weeks. Lice can otherwise persist in children's environments and reinfect them.

DOSAGE AND ADMINISTRATION

Thoroughly wash your child's hair with pyrethins shampoo as soon as you detect evidence of head lice. Use plastic gloves to apply the shampoo, and open the bathroom window to make sure the room is well-ventilated. Take care to apply only the amount recommended on the label, and leave on for ten minutes.

After washing, rinse thoroughly. Use a fine-toothed and

preferably disposable comb to remove any remaining head lice and their eggs from your child's scalp. Egg cases more than one-quarter inch from the scalp are not alive and do not need to be removed.

One thorough washing or rinse should be sufficient, as long as you are also certain to take appropriate measures to remove all lice from your child's environment. Pyrethins also have a residual effect that last for several weeks.

SIDE EFFECTS

Side effects due to treatment with pyrethins are uncommon. If your child develops a skin rash after treatment, consult your pediatrician.

IMPORTANT PRECAUTIONS

If your child is prone to allergic reactions of the skin, consult your pediatrician before using.

Pyrethins are not for internal use. If your child accidentally swallows any of the shampoo, call your poison control center.

Pyrethins should not be applied on open sores or wounds.

Take care that your child's eyes are protected from the shampoo. If shampoo accidentally enters eyes, immediately flush them with plenty of cold water.

Avoid inhaling the fumes of the shampoo.

SELENIUM SULFIDE

BRAND NAMES

Selsun, Selsun Blue

GENERAL INFORMATION

Selenium sulfide is the active ingredient in shampoo used to treat dandruff or seborrheic dermatitis of the scalp. It works by slowing the cell growth in scales on the scalp. Softened scales can be removed with a fine-toothed comb after the application of shampoo.

DOSAGE AND ADMINISTRATION

Wet your child's hair and scalp and apply the recommended amount of shampoo to form a lather. Rub in well, keeping away from eyes. Leave on three to five minutes, and rinse thoroughly.

The average use is twice a week. If no improvement is evident after two weeks, consult your child's pediatrician.

SIDE EFFECTS

Frequently occurring side effects due to treatment with selenium sulfide are uncommon.

Infrequent adverse reactions include dryness, itching, and rash. If your child experiences any of these effects, discontinue use and call your pediatrician.

IMPORTANT PRECAUTIONS

If your child is prone to allergic reactions of the skin, consult your pediatrician before using.

Selenium sulfide is not for internal use. If your child accidentally swallows any of the shampoo, call your poison control center.

Do not apply selenium sulfide to blistered or oozing skin.

Take care that your child's eyes are protected from the shampoo. If shampoo accidentally enters eyes, immediately flush them with plenty of cold water.

TOLNAFTATE

BRAND NAME

Tinactin

GENERAL INFORMATION

Tolnaftate is an antifungal medication used to fight fungal infections such as ringworm, athlete's foot, and jock itch. While fungal infections are not usually serious, their peeling and itching can make your child very uncomfortable. Tolnaftate works by damaging the cell walls of fungi and killing them.

DOSAGE AND ADMINISTRATION

Tolnaftate is available for children as a cream, lotion, ointment, or gel. If possible, wash and dry the affected area before applying medication.

Apply a thin coating to the affected area twice a day. The dosage is the same for all ages.

SIDE EFFECTS

No frequently occurring side effects are expected due to treatment with tolnaftate.

An infrequent adverse reaction is skin rash and irritation. If this occurs, discontinue use and consult your pediatrician.

IMPORTANT PRECAUTIONS

Tolnaftate should be used on children under two only under a pediatrician's supervision.

Tolnaftate is for external use only.

Cough and Cold Preparations

Viral respiratory infections affect children of all ages. Studies have shown that the normal, healthy preschool child can come down with as many as fifteen respiratory illnesses in one year. School-aged children also get lots of colds, although we don't exactly know how many. As a parent, you naturally want your sick child to feel as comfortable as possible during these periods. Some cold and cough remedies, along with medications for fever and aches and pains (acetaminophen or ibuprofen), can be valuable tools to help your child through these times. Others have little real value and may cause uncomfortable side effects.

There are basically four different types of drugs in cold and cough medicines. Antihistamines are supposed to dry up nasal secretions. Decongestants are intended to shrink swollen membranes, opening up nasal passageways. Expectorants loosen phlegm and help the cough lift it out of the bronchial tubes, while cough suppressants calm the tickle that leads to unnecessary coughs.

But do these remedies work? Everyone swears by their own remedy. Yet evidence of studies in older children and adults shows that decongestants are only somewhat effective and antihistamines have no effect on the majority of colds. Preschool children have rarely been studied, and the research that has been done suggests that antihistamines, decongestants, and expectorants have little effect on them.

In our office, we recommend acetaminophen or ibuprofen for fever and discomfort and, when necessary, dextromethorphan to suppress an unnecessary cough. We also suggest humidifiers and steam treatments. Rarely do we recommend antihistamines or decongestants for colds. In my opinion, a four- or five-drug treatment regimen is uncalled for (especially in preschool children). The truth is that runny noses and congestion don't bother most children, and the side effects of the medications far outweigh their usefulness in most situations.

I believe that parents should be careful not to overtreat a simple respiratory infection. Yet each parent can study the data we present here and make a decision about what is best for their own child. In the section that follows, we review in greater detail the various compounds used in cold and cough remedies. Detailed charts of the components of popular brand name products follow. Please keep in mind that individuals respond differently to colds, and a drug that works for one person may not provide any relief for another.

ANTIHISTAMINES

Antihistamines are drugs that block the effect of histamine, a substance released in allergy. The limited studies that have been done have shown a drying effect for chlorpheniramine (also known by the brand name Chlortrimeton), while no effect was shown for diphenhydramine (Benadryl) or triprolidine (in Actifed).

The antihistamines used in the remedies below are chlorpheniramine (by far the most popular antihistamine), diphenhydramine, brompheniramine, and triprolidine. They all share the same set of side effects, primarily drowsiness. Occasionally, an antihistamine will make a very young child "hyperactive" for a few hours. This effect diminishes as the child ages, but it is a good reason to avoid antihistamines (especially diphenhydramine) in children, especially preschoolers.

DECONGESTANTS

Decongestants are drugs that constrict blood vessels, thus reducing swelling. These drugs are not specific for the nose, and their side effects (nervousness, dizziness, rapid heart rate, and insomnia) vary a great deal from one child to another. Oral pseudoephedrine is the best-studied and the most commonly used. It has been shown to be effective in two studies involving school-age children. There is little difference between any of the decongestants and they can be considered interchangeable.

EXPECTORANTS

Only one expectorant, guaifenesin, is used in over-the-counter remedies for children. Studies of the drug have given conflicting results. Only one study of young children appears to be of acceptable quality. The study showed that patients thought that the phlegm in a productive cough was thinner and that the total amount of phlegm was reduced. There are no side effects. However, the use of expectorants is most likely of little importance.

COUGH SUPPRESSANTS

Dextromethorphan is a nonnarcotic cough suppressant that is very effective and has no noticeable side effects when given in usual doses. While it suppresses the cough caused by irritation, it will not suppress the cough required to clear phlegm. It is the only cough suppressant used in any of the remedies listed below. While codeine is an effective cough suppressant, it is not available without a prescription, and therefore is not a component of over-the-counter remedies.

COLD AND COUGH COMBINATIONS

As we have said, there are many different combinations that will treat any possible combination of symptoms. The parent's dilemma is which one, if any, to use. The choice must be tailored to each child's individual needs and responses. In addition, it can be argued that the side effects of drowsiness and/or excitability brought on by these drugs is worse than the disease itself. It may be just as effective to let the nose run free, if you can stand it, and let your child wear an old shirt to wipe his nose on. A study of one combination, using the ingredients in Dimetapp (an antihistamine and decongestant combination) showed that children who received medicine, a placebo, or no medicine at all felt the same relief of symptoms and improvement in the same amount of time.

One remedy that I emphatically *don't* recommend is a combination of multisymptom drugs with acetaminophen (Tylenol, Tempra, Panadol). While the combination itself does not pose a danger, many parents may not realize that acetaminophen is present and give a second dose of acetaminophen. These combinations therefore present potential hazards.

OTHER INGREDIENTS

In order for cough and cold medicines to be given to children they must be suspended in a liquid and made (somewhat) appealing. Many ingredients are used.

Sweeteners include sucrose (table sugar), sorbitol, and saccharine. Do not be fooled by claims for "sugar-free" syrups. "Sugar" in industry-speak is table sugar. Sorbitol, for example, is a sugar as well. Often saccharine, which laboratory studies have linked to bladder cancer in rats, is substituted. "Sugar-free" is a marketing ploy. Fortunately, no matter what sweetener is used, the quantity your child consumes is insignificant.

Artificial colors are a problem for some children. Most are not adequately tested. A listing of artificial colors used is on every label (if you look hard enough). Some new products are being made available dye-free.

Alcohol was a major ingredient of children's medicines for years. The word "elixir" technically means alcohol-based. However, recent improvements in manufacturing have made it possible to produce alcohol-free preparations. Now, most "elixirs" are alcohol-free.

The tables following page 243 list the brands of liquid cold and cough remedies that are commonly used for children. We have listed the active ingredients in each brand and noted whether they have alcohol or dye in them. It's important to pay careful attention to the frequency of administration. A drug that is given every four hours can mean twice as many power struggles with a resistant two-year-old as one that is given every eight hours, and the one medicine that is given every twelve hours, a cough suppressant, is very clearly the answer to many parents' medication difficulties. Many combination remedies achieve a lower frequency of dosage by simply increasing the quantity of medication per dose. This may work well, but keep in mind that it can also lead to more side effects.

With this information at your fingertips, you as a parent have the knowledge and power to make informed decisions about your child's treatment. Lastly, remember, no matter which of the remedies you choose, the cold will go away in a week. If it doesn't, consult your pediatrician.

O-T-C COLD AND COUGH REMEDIES

Brand	Subname	Antihistamine	Decongestant	Expectorant	Suppressant	Alcohol	Dye	Frequency/ Hours
Actifed	*Head Cold and Allergy*	Triprolidine	Pseudoephedrine			0	+	4 to 6
Benadryl	*Decongestant Elixir*	Diphenhydramine	Pseudoephedrine			+	+	4 to 6
Benadryl	*Elixir*	Diphenhydramine				0	+	4 to 6
Benylin	*DM*				Dextromethorphan	0	+	6 to 8
Delsym					Dextromethorphan	0	+	12
Dimetapp	*DM*	Brompheneramine	Phenylpropanolamine		Dextromethorphan	0	+	4
Dimetapp	*Elixir*	Brompheneramine	Phenylpropanolamine			0	+	4
Naldecon	*DX*		Phenylpropanolamine	Guaifenesin	Dextromethorphan	0	+	4
Naldecon	*EX*		Phenylpropanolamine	Guaifenesin		0	+	4
Novahistine	*DMX*		Pseudoephedrine	Guaifenesin	Dextromethorphan	+	+	4
Novahistine	*Elixir*	Chlorpheneramine	Phenylephrine			+	+	4
PediaCare	*Cough Cold*	Chlorpheneramine	Pseudoephedrine		Dextromethorphan	0	+	4 to 6
PediaCare	*Infants' Decongestant Drops*		Pseudoephedrine			0	+	4 to 6
PediaCare	*Night Rest*	Chlorpheneramine	Pseudoephedrine		Dextromethorphan	0	+	6 to 8

O-T-C COLD AND COUGH REMEDIES

Brand	Subname	Antihistamine	Decongestant	Expectorant	Suppressant	Alcohol	Dye	Frequency/ Hours
Robitussin	*CF*		Phenylpropanolamine	Guaifenesin	Dextromethorphan	0	+	4
Robitussin	*DM*			Guaifenesin	Dextromethorphan	0	+	4
Robitussin	*Expectorant*			Guaifenesin		0	+	4
Robitussin	*PE*		Pseudoephedrine	Guaifenesin		0	+	4
Robitussin	*Pediatric Cough*				Dextromethorphan	0	+	6 to 8
Robitussin	*Pediatric Cough & Cold*		Pseudoephedrine		Dextromethorphan	0	+	6
Robitussin	*Pediatric Night Relief*	Chlorpheneramine	Pseudoephedrine		Dextromethorphan	0	+	6
Sudafed	*Cough Syrup*		Pseudoephedrine	Guaifenesin	Dextromethorphan	+	+	4
Sudafed	*Syrup*		Pseudoephedrine			+	+	4
Triaminic	*AM Cough and Decongestant*		Pseudoephedrine		Dextromethorphan	0	0	6
Triaminic	*AM Decongestant*					0	NA	6
Triaminic	*DM*		Phenylpropanolamine		Dextromethorphan	0	+	4
Triaminic	*Expectorant*		Phenylpropanolamine	Guaifenesin		0	+	4
Triaminic	*Nite Lite*	Chlorpheneramine	Pseudoephedrine		Dextromethorphan	0	NA	6
Triaminic	*Sore Throat (1)*		Pseudoephedrine		Dextromethorphan	0	+	6

0 = No + = Yes

INDEX